WHAT TO DO ABOUT

WHAT TO DO ABOUT AIDS

Physicians and Mental Health Professionals
Discuss the Issues

Edited by

Leon McKusick

UNIVERSITY OF CALIFORNIA PRESS

Berkeley   Los Angeles   London

University of California Press
Berkeley and Los Angeles, California

University of California, Ltd.
London, England

Copyright © 1986 by The Regents of the University of California

Library of Congress Cataloging in Publication Data

What to do about AIDS.

   Papers from a conference convened in San Francisco Sept. 13–14, 1985 by the AIDS
Clinical Research Center at the University of California, San Francisco.
   Includes index.
   1. AIDS (Disease)—Psychological aspects—Congresses. I. McKusick, Leon.
II. University of California, San Francisco. AIDS Clinical Research Center.
[DNLM: 1. Acquired Immunodeficiency Syndrome—psychology—congresses.
WD 308 W555 1985]
RC607.A26W49 1987   616.97'92'0019   86-16189
ISBN 0-520-05935-2
ISBN 0-520-05936-0

2 3 4 5 6 7 8 9

Contents

Editor's Preface

Through its short and virulent history, AIDS has been seen as a gay disease by nongay people, as a disease of outcasts by those in the societal mainstream, as a problem of localities by the federal government, and as a problem of the United States by the world community. At the same time AIDS seems to stir everyone at a profound level, forcing us to ask probing questions about the interaction of health and lifestyle, the role of societal institutions, and even the value of life itself. Our understanding of human psychology tells us that the impact of AIDS is most probably strongest where it is most vehemently denied or blamed on someone else—whether the denial is on the part of those at risk, those that come into contact with those at risk, or even those who work for the governmental agencies charged with responding to health problems. We see good results with all these groups when the issue is confronted directly with information, when fears are aired, and when attitudes are challenged.

AIDS shows health professionals once again how intimate the links are among biological, behavioral, and social factors in the treatment of disease. Psychosocial factors influence susceptibility to AIDS, as well as the progression of the disease. The vital clinical role that mental health practitioners must play is being defined at several levels: when the individual is reacting to the threat of AIDS and shaping his behavior; when, after infection, the person is coping with the psychological effects and further adjusting his attitude toward treatment and health behavior; and when the person with AIDS is coping with the approach of death. We also need to intervene with those who have indirect experience of AIDS, where psychological factors are very much evident: in friends and relatives, and even health practitioners themselves. We have a responsibility to keep the community at large correctly and continually informed.

With these issues in mind, the AIDS Clinical Research Center at the University of California, San Francisco, convened a conference in San Francisco on September 13 and 14, 1985, which attracted a diverse audience of physicians, nurses, mental health professionals, and program administrators. The conference occurred at the time that actor Rock Hudson had come forward and helped the world acknowledge the problem of AIDS. As a result, we found that the conference audience also included concerned individuals, not previously associated with AIDS health issues, who were newly sensitized and mobilized to learn. The enthusiasm generated by this conference confirmed for us the existence of a dire need nationwide for education in specific medical, psychosocial, and policy aspects of AIDS.

The book is divided into four sections: First, basic medical information is provided, including neuropsychiatric developments. This information is accurate and up-to-date as of this publication, but the medical picture of AIDS continually changes. The information here should serve only as a background for readers who might then do more research in areas of specific interest. In order to stay informed, readers must continue to seek updates of medical developments.

Second, mental health aspects of the epidemic are described. The psychological picture of AIDS is less likely to change over time, because the threat of AIDS is similar to other psychological phenomena, and a body of knowledge from other disciplines about other problems can be adapted for use in interpreting AIDS psychosocial issues. The papers in the second section will be helpful as mental health practitioners adapt their own psychological approach to these issues. The information about populations affected by AIDS is extended to include information about how people cope with other life-threatening events.

In the third section, papers describe the specific impact of AIDS on various subgroups: gay men, drug users, newly seropositive individuals, women, and bereaved survivors.

Finally, because San Francisco had an early outbreak of this disease, the administrative strategies developed there were innovative attempts to serve the sudden and developing medical and psychosocial needs imposed by AIDS. In the fourth section, these efforts are described in the hope that others can learn from our successes and mistakes as we met the challenge of AIDS.

The authors of these papers are all people who have been psychologically affected by AIDS as well. As you read, you will be able to experience how these individuals integrate their own personal reactions with their professional opinions and factual information.

Everyone involved in the publication of this book is sensitive to the use of gender-specific pronouns. Because by far the largest at-risk and infected population with which this volume deals is that of gay men, the editors agreed at the outset generally to use the masculine form of pronouns where an impersonal singular pronoun is needed.

The papers could not have been published here without the fine editing of Jeanne Duell and fine transcribing work of Mary Goodell or the support of the Washington Research Institute, the San Francisco Department of Public Health, and the State of California Department of Health Services.

Thanks are given to those members of the conference faculty whose papers are not included here: Michael Gottlieb, M.D., UCLA; John L. Ziegler, M.D., UCSF; Tristano Palermino, M.S.W., San Francisco AIDS Foundation; Sam Picciotto, Ph.D., private practice, San Francisco; Dawn Cortland, R.N., M.P., UCSF; and Maureen O'Neill, M.S.W., Hospice of San Francisco. Also, we are deeply indebted to the support and direction of the individual and organizational members of the conference program committee: John L. Ziegler, M.D., Michael Gottlieb, M.D., John Fahey, M.D., Marcus Conant, M.D., Tim Wolfred, Ph.D., Helen Schietinger, M.A., R.N., James Dilley, M.D., Carole Migden, M.A., Jeannee Martin, R.N., M.P.H., Donald Catalano, M.S.W., Jeffrey Mandel, Ph.D., Sam Picciotto, Ph.D., Sally Martin, L.C.S.W., Cindi Dale, Sam Puckett, Steven Rogers, Don Abrams, M.D., Harry Hollander, M.D., Judy Macks, L.C.S.W., and Jackson Peyton.

Special thanks also to Jeffrey Amory, M.S.W., and Gary Titus, M.S.W., of the AIDS Activity Office of the San Francisco Department of Public Health, and to Kenneth Brock, M.S.W., of the California State Department of Health Services, for securing the grant that made this publication possible; to Lisa Capaldini, M.D., Tim Mess, M.D., and James Dilley, M.D., for reviewing the medical papers; to Dick Pabich, Michael Raines, and Cindi Dale for their invaluable extra help in organizing the conference on which this book is based.

Contributors

Donald I. Abrams, M.D., is assistant director of the AIDS Clinic at San Francisco General Hospital and assistant clinical professor of medicine and a member of the Cancer Research Institute at the University of California, San Francisco (UCSF). He is one of the leading experts on lymphadenopathy and AIDS-related conditions. He has lectured and presented on various aspects of the AIDS epidemic since its beginning as well as serving in an advisory capacity to public health organizations and agencies on medical and psychosocial issues.

John R. Acevedo, M.S.W., is psychiatric social worker for the UCSF AIDS Health Project and former epidemiological specialist for the Hawaii State Department of Health. Since 1974, he has served as a teacher and school director, and as a therapist with outpatient individuals, couples, and groups. His specialties have included VD control and substance abuse in addition to educational and mental health applications to high-risk populations for AIDS.

Marcus Conant, M.D., is the founder and former director of the AIDS Clinical Research Center at UCSF. He is clinical professor of dermatology at UCSF and in the private practice of dermatology. He founded the San Francisco AIDS Foundation and has served in several consultative, research, and educational positions throughout the epidemic.

Barbara G. Faltz, B.A., B.S.N., is coordinator of education for the UCSF AIDS Health Project. She has worked with substance abuse counseling and administration for the past eight years. She taught psychiatric nursing at Hayward Unified School District and worked for the Veterans Administration and private chemical dependency treatment programs.

Gayling Gee, R.N., M.S., has worked in public health nursing for ten years, more recently as charge nurse and acting head nurse at San Francisco General Hospital Adult Medical Clinic. She currently is head nurse of the Oncology/AIDS Clinic at SFGH.

Mark Gold, M.A., is coordinator of special projects for the UCSF AIDS Health Project. He is the former director of counseling in the San Francisco Department of Public Health's AIDS Antibody Testing Program. He has done research and clinical work in the field of cancer, drug addiction, and AIDS.

William Horstman, Ph.D., is a clinical psychologist in private practice in San Francisco, a diplomate in forensic psychology, and a member of the panel of expert witnesses of the Municipal Court. He has been treating the psychological sequelae of AIDS in gay men and medical practitioners since early in the epidemic.

Brookes Linton, M.S.W., is a medical social worker at San Francisco General Hospital.

Judy Macks, M.S.W., L.C.S.W., is mental health training coordinator and coordinator of services for persons with AIDS with the UCSF AIDS Health Project. She is also in private practice in San Francisco.

Leon McKusick, Ph.D., is adjunct assistant professor of medicine at UCSF, directing the AIDS Behavioral Research, Stress Reduction, and Mental Health Training projects. He also practices psychotherapy in San Francisco.

Scott Madover, M.A., M.F.C.C., has worked as a psychotherapist and clinical social worker in a number of settings, largely with substance abuse disorders. He is coordinator of drunk driving programs in San Francisco county and clinical social worker for the UCSF AIDS Health Project.

Jeffrey S. Mandel, M.P.H., Ph.D., is project director of the UCSF Biopsychosocial AIDS Project and a consultant to the UCSF AIDS Health Project. He has worked on projects related to AIDS since 1982 and practices psychotherapy in San Francisco.

Stephen Morin, Ph.D., is a clinical psychologist in private practice in San Francisco, assistant clinical professor of medicine at UCSF, and a consultant to several government agencies. He was cofounder of the Association of Lesbian and Gay Psychologists and, in 1973, president of the Society for the Study of Lesbian and Gay Issues. His research and writing have focused on the relationship between health beliefs and AIDS risk reduction. He currently is a member of the California AIDS Strategic Planning Commission and the California Council on Mental Health.

Sheila Namir, Ph.D., is director of the University of California, Los Angeles, Psychosocial AIDS Study and staff psychologist at UCLA Neuropsychiatric Institute and Hospital. She is codirector of the Separation and Loss Clinic at the Wright Institute in Los Angeles and project coordinator at UCLA of a program on the psychosocial aspects of cancer.

Lyn Paleo has worked at the San Francisco AIDS Foundation since May 1983. Currently, she is director of the Foundation's Northern California Services Department. She is also a member of the Women's AIDS Network and coauthored, with Laurie Hauer, R.N., the first AIDS educational material directed to women.

Jeffrey Sahl, Ph.D., is a clinical psychologist in private practice in San Francisco and a consultant to a large preschool system. He conducts the HIV groups for the UCSF AIDS Health Project. He is the former clinical director of IAL Adolescent Day Treatment Center in San Francisco.

Donald Sandner, M.D., is president of the Northern California Society of Jungian Analysts and has a private practice in San Francisco.

Helen Schietinger, R.N., M.A., formerly director of the Shanti AIDS Residence Program, is director of AIDS education, California Nursing Association. She has worked in the field of AIDS since December 1981, when she was Kaposi's Sarcoma Clinic Coordinator at UCSF. She has worked closely with the San Francisco Department of Public Health to develop services for people with AIDS. In 1985 she was invited by the Australian government to participate in a national conference and to consult with state health departments and local AIDS organizations.

Jerome Schofferman, M.D., is currently in private practice in San Francisco with a subspecialty of pain management, and has been medical director of Hospice of San Francisco since 1981. He served as assistant clinical professor of medicine at the UCLA School of Medicine. He has lectured extensively on pain and symptom management in the dying patient.

Neil Seymour, M.A., M.F.C.C., is coordinator of the AIDS Antibody Counseling Program at the UCSF AIDS Health Project, formerly supervising counselor with the Project's Alternative Test Site Counseling Program. He works with individuals and groups with AIDS-related concerns in his private practice in San Francisco.

Nancy Shaw, Ph.D., is director of Women's Programming at the San Francisco AIDS Foundation, taught at the University of California, Santa Cruz, and is currently visiting lecturer in social and behavioral sciences at the University of California San Francisco School of Nursing.

Paul Shearer, M.S.W., L.C.S.W., is in private practice in San Francisco and is affiliated with the hospice program at Garden Sullivan Hospital, Pacific Presbyterian Medical Center. He was instrumental in developing the counseling program on Ward 5B, the prototype AIDS unit at San Francisco General Hospital.

Mervyn F. Silverman, M.D., M.P.H., is president of the American Foundation for AIDS Research and program director of the AIDS Health Service Program of the Robert Wood Johnson Foundation. He was director of the San Francisco Department of Public Health, 1977–1985.

Samuel Tucker, M.D., M.P.H., is assistant clinical professor of psychiatry at UCSF and is medical director of Operation Concern at the Pacific Presbyterian Medical Center.

Daniel Turner, M.F.A., is enrolled in an M.S.W. program at San Francisco State University. He is a founding member of the board of the San Francisco AIDS Foundation and served on the board of the AIDS Action Council (also known as FARO, the Federation of AIDS-Related Organizations) until October 1985. He works at the San Francisco Human Rights Commission Lesbian Gay Advisory Committee on the issue of AIDS discrimination.

Paul Volberding, M.D., is chief of the AIDS activities and oncology divisions of San Francisco General Hospital. He helped organize the first and second international conferences on AIDS in 1985 and 1986, has served on numerous committees, and has presented in several educational forums since early in the epidemic.

Scott Wirth, Ph.D., is a clinical psychologist in private practice in San Francisco. From 1975 to 1980 he was on the staff of Operation Concern, Gay/Lesbian Counseling Services, Pacific Presbyterian Medical Center. He has lectured widely.

Deane L. Wolcott, M.D., is assistant professor in residence, Department of Psychiatry and Biobehavioral Sciences, UCLA School of Medicine, and associate chief, Consultation-Liaison Psychiatry Service, UCLA Neuropsychiatric Institute. He has worked clinically with and done research on a number of populations of seriously medically ill patients and authored and coauthored papers and research reports on psychosocial and psychiatric aspects of AIDS.

1

Introduction: What We Have Learned

MERVYN F. SILVERMAN

The history of medicine is replete with epidemics tragically affecting the lives of literally hundreds of thousands of individuals. I know of no disease over the last hundred years, however, that has been as complex as AIDS—acquired immunodeficiency syndrome—no disease that has so challenged the medical community, while at the same time raising seemingly insoluble problems of social morality and legality and creating ramifications that will be felt in our community as a result of our actions.

Now before looking back at the psychological and political climate of 1980 or 1981, we might just pick up a morning newspaper: "Policy on AIDS Students" is the banner headline on the front page. "Insurers Want To Require AIDS Tests" is on the second page. "One-third of San Francisco Tested for AIDS Positive," "French Youth Gets Heart from AIDS Victim." Those are on just the first two pages. The political cartoon on the editorial page is also relevant. An innocent little boy is standing over to one side holding his books, and on the other side is a woman with her hair sticking out in all directions, foaming at the mouth, screaming, jumping up and down. The caption reads, "Which can be transmitted by casual contact—AIDS or AIDS hysteria?" That says it all!

The increasing number of health practitioners involved in working with AIDS demonstrates commitment, concern, and dedication to a problem that is unique in modern medical history. Several years ago, when the disease was first becoming known, and manifesting itself primarily among gay men, the situation was complex. Opposing points of view, among both medical administrators and gay men, were being voiced. The gay community at that time was certainly frightened, but also upset that this disease was being called the "gay plague." As director of the public health department, I remember people asking me, "Can't we change that name?" I did not feel we would be too successful because the poor Legionnaires have named after them a disease that probably should have been named the Bellevue-Stratford disease after the hotel whose air conditioning spread the disease. My advisors began saying to me and others, "Listen, this is obviously not isolated in the gay community; no epidemic stays in one group. We ought to refer to this as a public health problem. Let's get away from considering it a gay disease." That made a lot of sense, and at many levels of government throughout the country, we tried to talk about it as a public health problem. Unfortunately, the money and the interest were not forthcoming from the federal government.

Men in the gay community then became angry at the lack of concern, stating, "Listen, this *is* a problem affecting gays. This is a gay problem; we need money for this disease."

These two views caused confusion in the general public. People were asking: "Gay disease—public health problem—gay disease—is it a problem for me?" Tremendous anxiety was generated in the gay community, but it subsided there before it did in the nongay community. One reason for that, which I think gets lost, is that gay men joined forces in many ways to work on this problem and provide information to their community.

Unfortunately, antagonism among gay groups was very bitter at that time, with vitriolic attacks against one another's stances toward AIDS: one view holding that gay men had moved through and were continuing with gay liberation, and did not approve of publicizing problems to do with sex on posters, on TV, in newspapers; and another view opposing this plea for silence, insisting that because people were dying, information had to be made public. After a great deal of rancor, various factions agreed to disagree. (The issues became moot anyway as many people realized that we needed to convey as much information as possible to help people avoid AIDS.) Such deeply felt convictions confirmed my sense that in terms of opinion there is no more a gay community than there is a nongay community. It is made up of people of all stripes and colors—conservative, liberal, and uninterested. So the word "community" is used for general distinctions.

Then there was the general community, where the anxiety level rose incredibly, especially in the summer of 1983. The phones at my office were ringing off the hook: "I work in the Court Clerk's office. Can I accept a piece of paper from someone who has AIDS?" "I'm having a swimming party, and I think a gay man may come to it. Is it safe to swim in the same pool?" "On a bus can I sit next to someone who has AIDS?" Such fears are what one hears around the country today, but they are no longer heard in San Francisco. There also was talk about the "innocent versus the guilty." Unfortunately, the media (and I think without malice) describes the "innocent transfusion victim" and then the homosexuals who are getting AIDS and spreading it. This view that homosexual victims of AIDS are guilty is not changing in many parts of the country.

Local government has been very responsive in San Francisco. The response has been positive from the Board of Supervisors and the mayor. The staff of the Department of Public Health, those who were there in 1981 and who are there now, has been superb trying to respond to this tragic problem. It must be emphasized that our response was made in conjunction with one from the gay community. In July 1981 we established a reporting system and a case registry for AIDS. Almost all the cases have been investigated, and interviewed whenever possible, with liaison established between the Department of Public Health and the various hospitals, private physicians' offices, the Centers for Disease Control, and many, many other groups. We had a lesbian and gay coordinating committee in the department, which I made departmentwide in 1979. That committee was ready and really hit the ground running to produce an early resource document, which was the first in the nation for providers of care and others, to give people some idea where to go and what would be done.

In October 1982 we established the multidisciplinary AIDS Clinic at San Francisco General Hospital, which opened three months later and involved screening, diagnosis, treatment, follow-up, education, and counseling. As the number of cases increased, other screening clinics were established throughout the city. The first inpatient unit was established in 1983. When I was first approached about setting this one up, I was a little reluctant. I felt that isolating patients would further give a leper-type connotation. I was persuaded otherwise, and it was probably the best persuasion I have had because it is an outstanding unit, considered the model around the country. When patients on the ward say, "I feel safe; I feel good," in the midst of the tragedy they are experiencing, it really demonstrates the quality of the unit.

The Department of Public Health also funded the counseling services in which both professional and paraprofessional practitioners worked with patients, with loved ones, and with the "Worried Well"—those in at-risk groups or not infected but with similar symptoms and concerned about their health. Since those early days, even more sophisticated programs have been established, including extended care services at Garden-Sullivan Hospital; home health care; social service advocacy and emergency housing, long-term housing; practical support for daily living, including transportation, shopping, cleaning, laundry, and other services. The emotional support and advocacy program at San Francisco General Hospital, with which the Shanti Project is very much involved, is another important service. Also funded is continuing substance abuse counseling for people with AIDS, with in-service training for the staff; mental health support at Ward 86, the out-patient unit; intervention services; psychological assessments; short-term treatment; educational support groups for AIDS patients; mental health and AIDS programs to train and support mental health professionals working with at-risk populations and with AIDS patients. Also very important are the youth outreach programs; San Francisco is probably one of the few areas where such services exist, in which we solicit referrals from youth service providers and offer individual consultation, health education, and in-service training.

I have noted more than once "in-service training," because I think it is very important that the people who are providing care be educated and kept updated about dealing with the issues as they face them. The AIDS Health Project provides psychological and general health assessments with special emphasis on the factors that reduce the immunity; what can be done to try to boost the immunity; organized facilitation of educational support groups focusing on stress, depression, prevention, sensible sex, and other issues.

I mention "sensible sex" because many commentaries are given on the impropriety of spending money to recommend it. They demonstrate the problem that we face. Political reaction also has occurred in Los Angeles with regard to a substance abuse pamphlet that was developed in San Francisco because it did not advocate total abstinence from drugs. It said, "If you're going to be using drugs, don't share needles." Unfortunately, that was not deemed moral enough. Some politicians were also upset by the brochure that I think has actually been quite good, called "Mother Knows Best," which was produced in Los Angeles. It is almost like a little Jewish mother telling her son to have "safe sex." Both have been taken off the market.

The issue that I think brings together all the moral, legal, and social aspects of AIDS is the bathhouse issue. When it became obvious that AIDS is a sexually transmitted disease and seemed associated with multiple anonymous contacts, it also became clear that bathhouses (and I use that term generically to include sex clubs as well) were facilitating such activity, and thus encouraging the spread of disease. But I became very much aware that these sites were not only buildings but represented what had taken place before liberation—they held historical significance for many in the gay community. Thus, it was not just a matter of closing a few buildings somewhere. They represented a refuge where gay men had been able to go in the past—a refuge for people who could not safely acknowledge their homosexuality in public. Therefore they had a great symbolic value. If government took that action, what would government do next? Would it close gay bars? Would sodomy laws be reinstituted, as was done in Texas in 1985?

I realized that the problem was basically a behavioral one. I felt that the public health department should, most usefully, work with the gay community to try to bring about changes in behavior. And by April 1984, changes in behavior had become significant. The rate of rectal gonorrhea had decreased 75 percent from 1980 to 1984, a fact that is rarely covered in the press. I know of no other situation in which that kind of change in behavior has ever been recorded. Take a hundred people who are overweight, put them on a diet, and what percentage end up losing weight and keeping it off? Less than 5 percent. Smoking? We all know the answer to that one. A 75 percent reduction in rectal gonorrhea represents an incredible change in behavior!

The 1984 figures were achieved largely through cooperation between the public health department and the community, with *great* work done by the AIDS Foundation and many, many other groups. At that point, it was decided to look at the bathhouse issue again. Only about 5 percent of the community was regularly going to the baths, but their use was still fostering the spread of a disease that the city was spending more than $6 million in 1984 to try to stop. It is somewhat like the issue of government subsidies for tobacco growers while the Department of Health and Human Services spends millions to try to convince people not to smoke the cigarettes that are supported by the Department of Agriculture.

I brought together an advisory group of twelve experts in a multidisciplinary approach—gay, nongay, state, federal, local—to discuss how we should approach the bathhouse use. I brought in a facilitator so I would not directly affect the process. There were many votes and many even divisions, but by the end, after six hours of exhausting debate, we reached a unanimous agreement as to what action should be taken.

At the time we did not yet have an etiologic agent, but there was good evidence that AIDS resulted from intimate body fluid exchange and susceptibility increased with multiple sexual partners. The discussion ranged around these issues, each of which had policy, legal, ethical, and civil rights considerations: Should the bathhouses be closed or should sex be limited within them? Was there enough medical information available to substantiate our position? Would closing them significantly alter behavior or would we simply cause a change in venue?

Would we lose an audience to whom we could distribute the necessary risk reduction information? Would a legal challenge reopen the baths immediately after we had closed them? Was it possible to prohibit fluid exchange without prohibiting sex in bathhouses? We discussed all the issues that were raised in public. We finally decided on the idea of using regulations so the owners of the establishments could improve their places, make structural changes, not allow the kind of behavior that would lead to the spread of the disease. Thus, they would have a chance to become acceptable from the health perspective.

I had hoped to have people from the gay community put pressure on the owners of bathhouses, but I was unsuccessful. In the 1970s, the community had taken action against gay bars that did not have two exits and were a fire hazard. Bars without the second exit were pick-eted by gay men until bar owners complied. But I could not convince anyone in the community to act. Some people who really did want the bathhouses closed explained that if the health department as a government agency closed the baths, they would protest and "man the barri-cades" because of the implications of that action. Instead, we drew up the regulations. The department promulgated them, and they were to be heard by the Police Department, which had that authority, but the hearing was canceled. There was a move on the Board of Supervisors to amend any action that was taken—regardless of where the authority rested—to say that the government could not regulate sexual activity. I thought this an unconscionable move because acts that arise from the Department of Public Health's ability to stem disease are appropriate. It would be similar to someone with positive feelings about toxic spills being able to interfere with the government's ability to stop those who are spilling toxins. Because of this political interference I reconvened the advisory group at the end of the summer. Whereas the first deci-sion had been unanimous, now there was a split: about half for closing the bathhouses, and the other half divided between waiting for the gay community to do something and voting not to close them at all.

I don't think anybody short of the bathhouse owners thought about bathhouses as much as I did, day and night for two years. And had I been on a debating team I could successfully have debated the issue on either side. Nevertheless, I decided that as a community we had reached a point at which we could no longer ignore the danger the bathhouses presented. I still had fears that ramifications from this action would spread across the nation. Nonetheless, millions were being spent to re-duce the spread of this disease and entrepreneurs were profiting from its spread. So I decided to close them. Having made the decision, I found it much easier to proceed and follow through:

Today I have ordered the closure of fourteen commercial establishments which promote and profit from the spread of AIDS—a sexually transmitted fatal disease. These businesses have been inspected on a number of occasions, and demonstrate a blatant disregard for the health of their patrons and of the community.

We now have solid evidence that AIDS is a sexually transmitted viral disease—often spread by people who are unaware that they are carrying the virus. Antibodies to this virus have been found in at least 40 to 50 percent of the gay male population studied in San Francisco. We know that the more sexual activity involving exchange of body fluids, the greater the risk of contracting AIDS.

From the beginning of this epidemic, we established a prevention program which placed major emphasis on education designed to inform the gay community about the nature of this disease and how it can be prevented. This became part of an overall approach by San Francisco that is serving as the model AIDS program for the rest of the country. Today's action is one part of this comprehensive program.

The places that I have ordered closed today have continued in the face of this epidemic to provide an environment that encourages and facilitates the multiple unsafe sexual contacts, which are an important factor in the spread of this deadly disease.

When activities are proven to be dangerous to the public and continue to take place in commercial settings, the health department has a duty to intercede and halt the operation of such businesses.

Make no mistake about it. These fourteen establishments are not fostering gay liberation. They are fostering disease and death. (October 9, 1984, S.F. Department of Public Health)

Later in October the city attorney and the public health department working together looked into about thirty locations, and in fourteen of them the spread of AIDS was being facilitated and encouraged. We closed them down, and they opened up the next day. We obtained a temporary restraining order and then a preliminary injunction, which was interesting because the judge ordered time be allowed to make structural changes in their establishments while prohibiting sexual activity, which was just what we had tried to do earlier, in April.

Looking back, I still believe it was the appropriate action to take at the time, considering the programs that were in place and the amount of money being spent. At that time we San Franciscans were far ahead of everyone else in the country in dealing with the whole issue of AIDS—and here it was appropriate. We had no illusions that the spread would end. We said we knew we would never even be able to document the impact the closings would have on the spread of the disease. But when I gave a talk to gay physicians in New York shortly after taking that action, I asked, "If there were no bathhouses and we were in the middle of the epidemic as we are right now, how many of you would support the opening of a bathhouse?" Not one hand was raised. And I think that pretty much sums up the issue. Again, I think the fact that government had to take the action represents a failure, just as any government intervention in one's personal activities represents a failure.

I was asked to say what I would do if I were the public health director of Laguna Beach, California, today. The first thought that jumped into my mind was, simply, resign. Actually, the answer is the answer to the title of this presentation—"What Have We Learned?" In a few words, it is *cooperate*, *coordinate*, and *educate*. And these should be done concurrently.

Government officials are the first group: Help them to understand what we health care providers and administrators are dealing with, what the issues are, and that we are not talking about morals or lifestyle. We are talking about an infectious agent. I find myself trying to explain why something is a sexually transmitted disease. I think people have an idea that some germs have prurient interests and just love to be involved in these activities. Of course, what it comes down to is that the virus is very fragile and therefore can be transmitted only this way. It is not something from a Stephen King movie coming over the horizon, gobbling up everything, and impossible to stop. Soap and water can kill the virus! So try to educate, to demonstrate that because it is fragile our children *can* go to school safely. That is also why we can sit on the bus or eat in the restaurant. I also tell people that there is probably no one, certainly in San Francisco, who has eaten in restaurants that has not been served at least once by someone who had gonorrhea at that time. Besides giving indigestion, this example causes people to realize that they do not get gonorrhea from eating in a restaurant. I think that puts AIDS, another sexually transmitted disease, in the proper perspective.

The second group is the gay community: Bring the people who are so deeply affected by AIDS into the planning, the programming, and the delivery of health care. The government has never been very good at trying to regulate "morality," and certainly attempts by government to control sexual activity have not been successful. I think the government should provide the funding and oversight and let the community do what it can do best, which is to relate to its constituents. It will be different in every community. In some, intravenous (IV) drug users are the largest group infected by AIDS. What we do in San Francisco probably would not be appropriate in Philadelphia or Chicago.

The next group is the media: Work with journalists in all aspects of the media to educate them. I think the press in San Francisco, with few exceptions, has been outstanding. But then one finds a headline writer who says "AIDS Jumps into the Heterosexual Community"—rather like a flea. Or one reads reports that AIDS may be passed in saliva because a seventy-four-year-old man who is diabetic, had lung cancer, had radiation and chemotherapy—and who therefore was "entitled" to have a compromised immune system—is assumed instead to have AIDS. If health care providers can work closely with the media, they help educate the people who really are undertaking the bulk of the education for the whole community.

Business leaders are another group. I spend a great deal of time with business leaders. They do not know how to deal with someone who returns to work with a diagnosis of AIDS or with someone who may have AIDS who applies for work. Should their concern be only with the confidentiality concerning the person coming back? What are their responsibilities to others on the staff? It is important to work with the business community, which might also help to get additional funding.

And, finally, the medical community: There are many confused people in the medical community. An infectious disease control physician in Bel Glade, Florida, says AIDS is spread by mosquitos. You know, that kind of statement goes all over the nation. And it increases fear and gives rise to calls for quarantine of persons with AIDS or even of those who have a positive result on the antibody test.

What have we learned? We have learned that education brings about prevention, which is the only defense we have against this disease. We do not have a vaccine; we do not have a cure. It must be prevention. And I think Thomas Adams summed it up very well about three hundred years ago when he said, "Prevention is so much better than healing because it saves the labor of being sick."

PART I

Medical Issues for Mental Health Practitioners

2

Issues of the Medical Treatment of AIDS Relevant to Mental Health Practitioners

DONALD I. ABRAMS

During a conference held in New York in February 1985, "AIDS in the Media," it was reported that San Francisco newspapers in 1984 had published the most stories in the country—140, compared with 50 published in New York City and 34 in Washington—about acquired immune deficiency syndrome (AIDS). More recently, however, syndicated columnists all over the country have looked at the AIDS problem: from Ann Landers to the venerable Gallup Poll. This increased public awareness and nationwide coverage is largely the result of the courage of the late Rock Hudson—one of Dr. Michael Gottlieb's now most famous patients in Los Angeles—in making public his AIDS diagnosis. I think it can be all too easy for San Francisco health care professionals and lay residents to learn too much of what we know about AIDS from the newspapers. That is probably why I always cherish the opportunity to talk to health care providers and health care professionals about what AIDS is and what AIDS is not, in order to share more of a firsthand view.

What Constitutes AIDS?

AIDS, as defined by the Centers for Disease Control (CDC), is the presence of a reliably diagnosed disease that is at least moderately indicative of underlying cellular immunodeficiency in a person without underlying immune deficiency state, on no medications that are known to cause immune suppression, and with no underlying malignancy, such as lymphoma, which can cause immunosuppression.

There is a multitude of different diagnoses for AIDS (Allen 1984, Fauci et al. 1984, Fauci et al. 1985, Gottlieb et al. 1983). Far and away the most common diagnosis is the infection *Pneumocystis carinii* pneumonia (Gottlieb et al. 1981). Pneumocystis pneumonia is not a new disease, although it is relatively new in the history of medicine. First described in starving European children after World War II, it is caused by an amoeba. Most of us have been exposed to this amoeba at some time in our childhood because by the time we are four years old the majority of us have antibodies to the pneumocystis organism. It usually does not cause disease because our immune systems are intact. Only when the immune system is destroyed does this organism, as well as most of the other organisms, have the opportunity to cause infection. Thus, they are called "opportunistic" infections. *Pneumocystis carinii* pneumonia accounts for more than 50 percent of all the AIDS diagnoses in the United States.

Toxoplasma gondii is another amoebic organism. This organism is found in cat feces, which is why pregnant women are advised not to handle cat litter boxes. In some populations, toxoplasma causes an illness like mononucleosis, with swollen glands, fevers, and fatigue. In AIDS patients, however, toxoplasma causes abscesses in the brain; thus, clearly it is an illness in which patients might present with some neuropsychological manifestations (Luft et al. 1984). *Cryptosporidium* is another infecting protozoan, which causes a profound diarrhea in AIDS patients, who may have up to five liters of watery stool a day. Usually occurring in the terminal stages of the illness, the uncontrollable diarrhea is very debilitating and distressing for dying patients, already quite wasted from the ravages of their disease.

The fungal infections that constitute an AIDS diagnosis include *candida*, the yeast that often causes vaginitis in women, especially after antibiotic therapy. In our patients, to constitute an AIDS diagnosis, candida must infect the esophagus or be disseminated throughout the body. Many patients in risk groups in San Francisco have a yeast infection of the mouth, oral candida, or thrush. Although this does indicate the presence of underlying defects in the immune system, oral candida does not in and of itself constitute an AIDS diagnosis, which requires at least involvement of the esophagus.

Cryptococcus is another organism that has a reservoir in animals—it is usually found in pigeon droppings. Cryptococcal meningitis has been a disease seen in other immunocompromised patients, predominantly patients receiving chemotherapy for lymphoma or leukemia. In AIDS patients we see not only cryptococcal meningitis, which certainly can present with central nervous system manifestations, but also cryptococcal sepsis.

The bacterial infections that constitute an AIDS diagnosis are not the traditional staph and strep or gram-negative rods that one would expect to see in immunocompromised patients. Our most common bacterial infection is actually an atypical mycobacterium, in the same family as tuberculosis, *mycobacterium avium-intracellulare* (Mess et al. 1985). As you can see from the root word "avium," this organism also has a reservoir in the bird population. In contrast to tuberculosis, which is a readily treatable infection today, *mycobacterium avium-intracellulare* unfortunately is exquisitely resistant to all antibiotics. We have been treating our patients with up to five different antibiotics with quite a bit of toxicity and not too much efficacy. A 1985 report by the group from Memorial Sloan-Kettering Cancer Center in New York City described their response in treating large numbers of patients with this mycobacterium (Hawkins et al. 1985). Comparing patients who had been treated to a group who had not, they found at autopsy that those patients who had been treated for the infection actually had more disseminated disease than those who had not. Perhaps the patients whom they elected to treat had more disseminated disease at the beginning. We need to reevaluate what exactly to do when we discover this infection in our patients.

The viral infections that constitute an AIDS diagnosis include chronic mucocutaneous herpes simplex. Most commonly what we see are herpes lesions around the anal region that do not heal. Cytomegalovirus (CMV), another virus in the herpes family, in many people causes an asymptomatic infection or a mild mononucleosislike picture, perhaps with some hepatitis. For AIDS to be diagnosed on the basis of CMV infection alone, organs other than the lymph nodes or the liver must be involved. We most often see CMV infection of the retina, causing blindness. We also see CMV pneumonia, as well as colitis and possibly encephalitis.

Progressive multifocal leukoencephalopathy (PML) is an unusual central nervous system infection—a dementing, debilitating illness, in which patients gradually, or sometimes not so gradually, progress to a vegetative state (Blum et al. 1985). This infection is felt to be caused by a papovavirus. Now that we are learning more about the AIDS virus, I wonder if PML actually is an AIDS-related diagnosis. What we might really be seeing is, in fact, central nervous infection with the AIDS virus itself.

The malignancies that constitute an AIDS diagnosis are Kaposi's sarcoma (KS), primary central nervous system lymphomas, and peripheral non-Hodgkin's lymphomas in the presence of a positive antibody to the AIDS virus.

Those of us who have been working in the field for some time, however, realize that the surveillance definition and this list of opportunistic infections and malignancies are just what was very obvious at the beginning of the epidemic in 1981. Similar to the reactions to hepatitis B, not everybody who is infected with the virus has the same manifestations of the disease. With hepatitis B some people become infected and die very rapidly of fulminent liver failure; some turn yellow and get hepatitis; some get hepatitis and do not turn yellow; some become asymptomatic carriers of hepatitis B; some make antibodies and become immune. I think that such is the case with infection by the AIDS virus. Not everyone infected reacts the same way. What we have recognized is a large group of persons that forms the base of the so-called AIDS iceberg, those who have AIDS-related conditions (ARC), but whose symptoms do not constitute a diagnosis of AIDS.

The other malignancies that we have seen with increased frequency in the at-risk population in San Francisco include, as I mentioned, the non-Hodgkin's lymphoma as well as Hodgkin's disease. Other clinicians have reported an increased incidence of squamous cell carcinoma of the tongue and the rectum.

Persistent unexplained lymphadenopathy, or swollen glands, is an area of my particular interest. A large group of persons in AIDS risk populations is expressing infection with the AIDS virus by the presence of this condition, which will be discussed below (Laurence et al. 1984). Similarly, idiopathic or immune thrombocytopenic purpura (ITP)—a condition of low platelet counts that may lead to life-threatening bleeding, more commonly seen in young children or middle-aged women—has also been reported to be affecting those in the AIDS risk groups (Abrams et al. 1986). In 1985, in our clinic at San Francisco General Hospital, we were following forty men with ITP. The difficulty is that the treatment normally calls for steroids, which are further immunosuppressing, or for removing the spleen. This has been, therefore, a particularly challenging problem.

The Immune System Problem in AIDS

All the different disorders on the iceberg, both at the tip and the base, have an underlying theme that unites them—immune dysfunction.

Our immune system is built up of a channel, the communication of the lymphatics, the lymph vessels, and the lymph nodes throughout the body. The spleen is another major organ of the immune system. It acts largely as an enlarged lymph node to house the lymphocytes, or the building-block blood cells of the immune system. The thymus is an important gland that overlies our heart, but that usually involutes by the age of five. By the time it does involute, however, it has pro-grammed all the T-lymphocytes that we need for life. It perhaps con-tinues to produce thymic hormones, however, throughout our lives.

The immune response is the body's primary defense against foreign invaders. When a foreign protein, or antigen, enters the body, it is pro-cessed by the scavenger cell, the so-called monocyte/macrophage. The foreign protein, or antigen, is then presented to our lymphocytes so that they can respond appropriately. We have two major families of lymphocytes: B-cells, which respond by producing an antibody to neutralize the foreign invader, and T-cells, which go out and ingest the foreign invader itself by cell-mediated immunity, not by produc-ing the antibody, that is, not by humoral immunity.

In the T-cell family we have two subsets, the helper T-cell and the suppressor T-cell. They do what their names imply. Helper T-cells are important to boost and augment the function of the entire immune system. We can think of the helper T-cell as the orchestra leader of the entire immune response. The suppressor cell acts at the end of the pro-cess. When the virus is gone, and we need not respond to it anymore, suppressors turn off the immune response. Normally, healthy people have twice as many helper T-lymphocytes as suppressor T-lympho-cytes. The problem in AIDS is a disappearance or depletion of the helper T-cell population.

For a long time we were not sure what was causing this. Even before we identified the AIDS retrovirus we were pretty certain that it was a response to a viral infection. This virus has been called human T-cell lymphotropic virus type III (HTLV-III), or lymphadenopathy-associated virus (LAV), or AIDS-related virus (ARV): three names for the same virus.* Now we know that this virus infects the helper T-lymphocyte, leading to its death and destruction, allowing the im-mune response to become haywire, and opening up the door for the development of the opportunistic infections and malignancies. Basi-cally, that is what causes AIDS.

Retrovirus Activity in the Body

HIV belongs to a unique family of viruses. A virus is a piece of genetic information, either DNA or RNA, surrounded by a protein coat that

---

*A subcommittee of the International Committee on the Taxonomy of Viruses in 1986 recommended that the AIDS retrovirus be called *human immunodeficiency virus,* or *HIV.* The usage has been adopted in this volume to replace the several designations of the AIDS virus described above that have been previously used. (Editor) protects it from the environment. Retroviruses are very small viruses composed of a single strand of RNA, the intermediate nucleic acid in the production of proteins. Normally, the flow of genetic information starts with a piece of DNA, which makes a piece of RNA, which in turn codes for protein. Everything flows in that direction. Retroviruses contain a unique enzyme called reverse transcriptase, which allows this single strand of RNA, that is, the virus, to make itself *back* into a piece of DNA, going backward against the flow of genetic information. Hence, "retrovirus." This piece of viral DNA then inserts itself into the genetic material of the cell that it is infecting, in this case the helper T-lymphocyte, and it remains intertwined there for the life of the cell.

Retroviruses are not unique to man; in fact, they have been only relatively recently described in man. In 1980, the first retroviral disease in humans was recognized, adult T-cell leukemia lymphoma, a very aggressive form of lymphoma caused by the virus called human T-cell leukemia virus type I (HTLV-I) and found in the southern islands of Japan. Retroviruses, however, have been found and identified in lower animal species since the beginning of this century. Perhaps the most widely known retrovirus is feline leukemia virus. Retroviruses work in other animals similarly to the way they proceed in AIDS, causing prolonged immune suppression by infecting a subclass of lymphocytes. In AIDS it is the helper T-cell that we think is the predominant target of the infection.

Since the retrovirus does live in the lymphocyte, which is a blood cell, it makes sense that it can in fact be cultured from the blood, the bone marrow, and the lymph nodes. The retrovirus, however, does not need the cells. It has also been found in cell-free plasma, as well as in saliva. Semen is a very potent source of the retrovirus, probably because there are multiple lymphocytes present in the seminal ejaculate.

The significance, however, of finding HIV in these various secretions remains uncertain. A much-publicized event in Sacramento, California, highlights that. The sheriff said that mouth-to-mouth resuscitation should not be performed on gay men because of the possibility of transmitting the retrovirus. When a news team from Sacramento interviewed me, I looked right at the camera and said, "I'd like to ask the sheriff of Sacramento a question. Suppose he needed CPR and the only person around to give it to him was a gay man. Would he then be so concerned about transmission of this disease?"

Headlines have proclaimed film and television actresses' fear of kissing male actors; news reports have mentioned tears and sweat. I think that HIV will be found in many secretions. This, however, does not change our understanding of how the disease is *transmitted*. AIDS is transmitted through intimate sexual contact with exchange of body fluids and also through contaminated blood products. I do not know of many diseases that are transmitted through tears, and there are no documented cases of AIDS in which saliva was the transmitting fluid.

In addition to infecting the helper T-lymphocyte, the virus also, according to evidence, infects cells of the central nervous system, that is, the brain (Jordan et al. 1985, Levy et al. 1985; chapter by Wolcott below). We noticed in doing head computed tomography (CT) scans on a number of our patients, even before we knew what caused this disease, that often reports showed marked cortical atrophy. What we saw were enlarged ventricles and deepened sulci on the CT scan, suggesting that the patients, mainly in their twenties or thirties, have brains that look like those of people in their sixties or seventies. The cause for this was unknown.

Again, the group from Memorial Sloan-Kettering Cancer Center reported in Atlanta, in April 1985, on their experience doing autopsies on the brains of AIDS patients. Out of 106 brains they found only 6 that were entirely normal. One-third of them had space-occupying lesions, two-thirds of them had diffuse disease. Microscopic investigation suggested that the problem in the brains was a viral infection. In some cases they thought it might be CMV encephalitis, but in the majority they felt that the most obvious and likely cause was infection of the brain with HIV itself. I think this picture and much of what we used to call PML probably are secondary to HIV infecting the central nervous system. This is a big problem with regard to therapy, certainly, because not many medications that we currently use are able to cross the blood/brain barrier.

Disease Development and Treatment

Often we see patients who clinically appear to have something amiss in their central nervous system but with a negative head CT scan. At San Francisco General Hospital, we repeat the scan in time if we have a high index of suspicion. Unfortunately we do not have magnetic resonance imaging (MRI), which gives better resolution and is more sensitive in AIDS than routine CT scanning. One patient continued to have subtle changes in mental status as noted by his roommates. He had a negative CT scan on March 2, 1985. When it was repeated on April 4, lesions characteristic of toxoplasmosis were seen. The lesions were found in the internal capsule, again characteristic of toxoplasma abscesses. Interestingly, although these two masses in the brain look ominous, one month later they both disappeared after the patient was treated with sulfadiazine and pyrimethamine. Thus, this is one of the infections that can be treated with some effect, although lifelong maintenance therapy may be necessary.

KS has been the most common AIDS-associated malignancy (Mitsuyasu et al. 1985). The lesions it causes are violaceous; they do not itch, they do not hurt, they often are slightly raised. KS was previously recognized in elderly Italian and Jewish men, in whom the lesions were confined predominantly to the lower extremities. Unfortunately, however, in the AIDS patients the lesions are not thus restricted; they are diffused over the body. Facial lesions are particularly frustrating and demoralizing because clearly they mark the person as having AIDS, and they are easily recognized by the public.

As a malignancy of the lymphatic endothelium, KS often gives patients marked edema, or swelling, before the lesions appear. Patients with marked edema, either of the face or the extremities, may get some palliation from radiation therapy. At San Francisco General Hospital many methods have been used to treat KS. We have used chemotherapy with some success; regimens including single agents, predominantly vinblastine, or vinblastine alternating with vincristine, have been effective in about 30 percent of patients treated.

In an effort to reverse some of the immune suppression in our KS patients, we tried some immunomodulatory therapy with alpha interferon. We achieved approximately 40 percent responses, either complete or partial, but at the expense of producing more symptoms than the weekly chemotherapy provided. Gamma interferon and interleukin-2 are two other immunomodulators that we have used, but KS progressed with those treatments and no immune reconstitution has been apparent.

The current more rational therapy that we are attempting is antiviral therapy. At San Francisco General, we conducted a protocol with suramin, a reverse transcriptase inhibitor, and a study with HPA-23, the drug that the French have used. The reporting on both of these drugs is that in a small number of patients, but certainly not all patients, the virus is eliminated from the person's body. But the KS continues to progress. I think that by the time a person has AIDS and KS, the virus has already devastated the immune system to the point where antiviral therapy is probably not going to work alone.

Most of our patients with KS develop an opportunistic infection. Patients who have KS in the lungs generally in our experience have a life span of two months after the pulmonary diagnosis. A subset of patients with no opportunistic infections, who have minimal disease, can live for up to three or four years without therapy (Krigel et al.

1985). Another subset of patients, however, goes through a very disturbing, wasting illness at the end, with fevers, diarrhea, and loss of weight. They ultimately die of inanition.

Like toxoplasmosis, pneumocystis is a treatable infection, using either septra or pentamidine. We are also investigating the use of other drugs as well. The pneumocystis infection can be eradicated or clinically improved after two or three weeks of treatment. Patients with pneumocystis are, however, subsequently at risk for other opportunistic infections after treatment. The life span of a patient with pneumocystis has not been increased over the past five years of treatment in San Francisco, with our average life span remaining 9.6 months after diagnosis. So, although it is an infection, pneumocystis, interestingly and paradoxically, carries a worse prognosis than the malignancy KS.

Another severe, psychologically upsetting problem often seen in our patients with opportunistic infections, especially terminal patients, is the development of CMV retinitis. Destruction of the retina occurs through hemorrhage and exudates. Patients of mine who had KS for years developed pneumocystis and lived through that. Two years later they suddenly became blind. They felt they had really had enough when their sight was taken away. The infection is definitely debilitating and terribly demoralizing. An experimental drug, DHPG, is showing some effectiveness in stopping the progress of CMV retinitis.

AIDS-Related Complex

Describing patients with the so-called AIDS-related complex or condition (ARC) is describing a number of different patient populations. In this, it is similar to AIDS itself, which is an umbrella definition under which many subdiagnoses are included. Generally, when talking about ARC patients, we mean those who have constitutional symptoms, laboratory abnormalities, usually enlarged lymph nodes, all very suggestive of, or definitely indicating having been infected with HIV. But when we talk about ARC patients we really need to be more specific in order to know their natural history. A large number of patients with ARC have the so-called persistent generalized lymphadenopathy syndrome. Some ARC patients actually have a frank AIDS prodrome. We know that they are on their way to getting AIDS; they just do not have it yet. Other ARC patients are those who have a chronic wasting syndrome and die of severe manifestations of ARC, without ever developing an AIDS diagnosis. Some of the patients diagnosed with ARC probably do have an acute AIDS diagnosis.

The lymphadenopathy syndrome has been my main research concern (Abrams 1985, Abrams 1986). Patients may have bulky, visible lymphadenopathy, which is stressful for them despite biopsies showing the condition to be a benign reactive lymph node enlargement. They find it very difficult to accept. They wake up every morning reminded that they do have this evidence of infection with HIV, uncertain what their natural history might be.

Lymphadenopathy patients are prone to numerous minor infections that are not life threatening. These include skin fungal infections, herpes simplex and zoster, oral candida, and viral hairy leukoplakia, recurrent pharyngitis, and intestinal parasites. They may also have psychological problems of debilitating anxiety and depression. Patients with ARC, with lymphadenopathy, are in a large gray zone. They do not know if they will stay with lymphadenopathy for the rest of their lives or if they are at risk to develop AIDS. This deeply affects their ability to function in society. At one point, we did form a support group for patients with lymphadenopathy syndrome. But it had to disband after about five months because the rampant anxiety and depression within it was unconquerable.

The natural history of the 200 men that we have been following with persistent generalized lymphadenopathy since 1981 suggests that 10 percent of our patients, or 20 out of 200 men, progressed from 1981 to 1985 from lymphadenopathy to a bona fide AIDS diagnosis. In studying the problem, we still have not had enough time to know what the ultimate number of patients progressing will be.

We have tried to stop this progress in some patients whom we feel to be at greater risk. At San Francisco General Hospital we have done three studies of agents including alpha interferon, isoprinosine, and suramin to see which, if any, decrease the symptoms of the lymphadenopathy patients and prevent them from developing AIDS.

Precautions and Attitudes of Health Practitioners

Because of the fear that may be generated in working with AIDS patients, in conclusion I want to recapitulate important infection-control precautions. Careful handwashing and hepatitis B precautions are adequate.

In contrast, physicians during another epidemic in the history of medicine felt a need to protect themselves further. During the plague in the fourteenth century in Italy, physicians caring for the afflicted did not get the disease. Their outfit was made completely of leather, from the hood down to the floor. It had a wide-brimmed hat, which kept the doctor distant from the patient. In a large beak worn on the face, also to keep him at a distance from the patient, were stored herbs to keep the air clean. The doctors never touched the patients with their hands; they used a stick. Interestingly, the religious people, the monks, caring for plague patients without benefit of this protective barrier got the plague, but the doctors did not. That is because the plague is transmitted by fleas. AIDS is not. AIDS is transmitted through sexual contact with exchange of genital secretions and by contaminated blood products. I believe that wearing an outfit like that or even donning psychic armor that suggests this sort of barrier serves only to increase the social isolation and alienation that our patients already feel as a result of their diagnosis.

References

Abrams, D. I. 1985. Lymphadenopathy syndrome in male homosexuals. In *Advances in host defense mechanisms*, ed. J. I. Gallin and A. J. Fauci, pp. 75–97. New York: Raven Press.

Abrams, D. I., D. D. Kiprov, J. J. Goedert, et al. 1986. Antibodies to human T-lymphotropic virus type III and development of the acquired immunodeficiency syndrome in homosexual men presenting with immune thrombocytopenia. *Ann Int Med* 104:47–50.

Abrams, D. I. 1986. Lymphadenopathy related to the acquired immunodeficiency syndrome in homosexual men. *Med Clin of No Amer* 70:693–706.

Abrams, D. I., J. W. Dilley, L. M. Maxey, P. A. Volberding. 1986. Routine care and psychosocial support of the patient with the acquired immunodeficiency syndrome. *Med Clin of No Amer* 70:707–20.

Allen, J. R. 1984. Epidemiology of the acquired immunodeficiency syndrome (AIDS) in the United States. *Semin Oncol* 11:4.

Blum, L. W., R. A. Chambers, R. J. Schwartzman, et al. 1985. Progressive multifocal leukoencephalopathy in acquired immune deficiency syndrome. *Arch Neurol* 42:137.

Britton, C. B., and J. R. Miller. 1984. Neurologic complications in acquired immunodeficiency syndrome (AIDS). *Neurol Clin* 2:315.

Fauci, A. S., A. M. Macher, D. L. Longo, et al. 1984. Acquired immunodeficiency syndrome: Epidemiologic, clinical, immunologic, and therapeutic
considerations. *Ann Int Med* 100:92–106.

Fauci, A. S., H. Masur, E. P. Gelmann, et al. 1985. The acquired immunodeficiency syndrome: An update. *Ann Int Med* 102:800–13.

Gottlieb, M. S., J. E. Groopman, W. M. Weinstein, et al. 1983. The acquired
immunodeficiency syndrome. *Ann Int Med* 99:208.

Gottlieb, M. S., R. Schroff, H. M. Schanker, et al. 1981. *Pneumocystis carinii*
pneumonia and mucosal candidiasis in previously healthy homosexual men:
Evidence of a new acquired cellular immunodeficiency. *N Engl J Med* 305:
1425–31.

Hardy, A. M., J. R. Allen, W. M. Morgan, et al. 1985. The incidence rate of
acquired immunodeficiency syndrome in selected populations. *JAMA*
253:215.

Hawkins, C., T. E. Kiehn, E. Whimbey, et al. 1985. Treatment of *M. avium-
intracellulare* infection in AIDS. In *Proceedings of the international conference on
AIDS*, p. 49. Atlanta, Georgia.

Jordan, B., B. A. Navia, S. Cho, et al. 1985. Neurological complications of
AIDS: An overview based on 110 autopsied patients. (abstract) In *Proceedings of the international conference on AIDS*, p. 49. Atlanta, Georgia.

Krigel, R., R. Ostreicher, F. LaFleur, et al. 1985. Epidemic Kaposi's sarcoma
(EKS): Identification of a subset of patients with a good prognosis. *Proc Am
Soc Clin Oncol* 4:4.

Laurence, J., F. Brun-Vezinet, S. E. Schutzer, et al. 1984. Lymphadenopathy-
associated viral antibody in AIDS. *N Engl J Med* 311:1269.

Levy, R. M., D. E. Bredesen, M. L. Rosenblum. 1985. Neurological manifestations of the acquired immunodeficiency syndrome (AIDS): Experience
at UCSF and review of the literature. *J Neurosurg* 62:475–95.

Luft, B. J., R. B. Brooks, F. K. Conley, et al. 1984. Toxoplasmic encephalitis in patients with acquired immune deficiency syndrome. *JAMA* 252:
913–17.

Mess, T. P., W. K. Hadley, and C. B. Wofsy. 1985. Bacterimia due to *Mycobacterium tuberculosis* (MTB) and *Mycobacterium avium intracellulare* (MAI) in ho-

mosexual males. In *Proceedings of the international conference on AIDS*, p. 47. Atlanta, Georgia.

Mitsuyasu, R., R. Afrasiabi, J. Taylor, et al. 1985. Immunologic prognostic variable in patients with AIDS and Kaposi's sarcoma (KS). (abstract) *Proc Am Soc Clin Oncol* 4:1.

Nielsen, S. L., C. K. Petito, C. D. Urmacher, et al. 1984. Subacute encephalitis in acquired immune deficiency syndrome: A postmortem study. *Am J Clin Pathol* 82:678–82.

Shaw, G. M., M. E. Harper, B. H. Hahn, et al. 1985. HTLV-III infection in brains of children and adults with AIDS encephalopathy. *Science* 227: 177–82.

Valle, S.-L., C. Saxinger, A. Ranki, et al. 1985. Diversity of clinical spectrum of HTLV-III infection. *Lancet* 1:301–4.

Volberding, P. A. 1985. The clinical spectrum of AIDS—implications for comprehensive patient care. *Ann Int Med* 103:729–33.

3

Questions from Mental Health Practitioners About AIDS

MARCUS CONANT

When the experts say that AIDS is not transmitted by casual contact, what do they mean? Is it transmitted like other viruses?

Viruses are generally transmitted through body secretions—saliva, semen, blood, urine, feces—or through the respiratory system from small droplets when an individual coughs. You don't have to kiss someone to catch the flu from him; simply being in a room and breathing the same air contaminated with infectious virus will suffice. No one has contracted AIDS in this manner. The message that we need to proclaim over and over and over again is: To contract this disease you must receive blood from an individual who is infected, share a needle that is contaminated with blood from that individual, or have unsafe sex with that individual.

While taking care not to make the patient feel like a leper, what precautions should nurses and hospital personnel take to avoid infection from someone who has AIDS? Where is more information available?

The shortest answer for hospital personnel is that they should care for patients infected with HIV and handle blood and secretions from those patients in exactly the same way that they were taught to care for patients who are infected with hepatitis B. The San Francisco AIDS Foundation has put together an excellent brochure on infection control guidelines, which is available from the foundation.

As a health care practitioner, I have a client who continues to have high-risk sex that in my mind would transmit the AIDS virus. What information should I give this person?

This raises a number of important questions. From the bloodstream of individuals who are infected or who are antibody-positive, live virus is recovered 60 to 80 percent of the time. It is not yet clear whether this means that there are periods with no active virus, indicating that the person's own resistance is containing the infection, or whether the culture techniques are just so insensitive that we do not get 100 percent recovery.

Virus recovery in 70 to 80 percent of infected men leads me to believe that somewhere in the neighborhood of 75 percent of men who are antibody-positive are also shedding virus intermittently. You therefore have the clear obligation to counsel your patient that he *is* infected with HIV and, in all likelihood, is shedding active virus in his semen that could infect his sexual partner. "Safe sex," or non–body-fluid exchange sex should be employed 100 percent of the time. Men should disclose their antibody positivity and the facts just enumerated to their sexual partners so that the latter may make an informed decision as to whether they wish to place themselves at risk of infection with a potentially fatal disease.

What about AIDS in other countries? Is it transmitted any differently in Africa or Europe?

In the United States, the vast majority, 98 percent of AIDS patients, are men and only 2 percent or so are women. (These are 1985 percentages. The figures are changing rapidly.) In Haiti it would look as if the figures are 60 percent men, 40 percent women. There is evidence in this country that HIV is easily spread from a man to another man or from a man to a woman, even if they do not have rectal sex. Rectal sex may be the primary way of transmission between men; but I know of some women who have had only vaginal sex with men who have become infected with HIV. So transmission from man to man and man to woman can be documented. There is also documentation of transmission of the virus from woman to man.

What medical reasons would prompt taking the HIV antibody test?

Clearly, donors who plan to give corneas or kidneys or hearts for organ transplantation or who plan to donate semen for artificial insemination and individuals planning to give blood for use in transfusions need to be antibody tested to see if their organs or blood have been infected with the AIDS retrovirus. This is so necessary that donors are not asked the results of their test, rather they are informed that the testing *will be done*. After the organ is taken or before the blood is used for transfusion, it is tested to see that it is HIV negative. Women contemplating pregnancy need to consider whether they are positive or negative. If you have a two-thirds chance that your newborn child will be infected with HIV and develop AIDS and die, you may give serious consideration to avoiding pregnancy or having a therapeutic abortion if you have become pregnant. These considerations are no longer theoretical. Blood banks are testing every unit of blood for HIV antibody; pregnant women are being counseled about risk.

Individuals (suspecting they *may* have been infected with HIV) who plan to have an ongoing sexual relationship without being able to practice safe sex 100 percent of the time should be urged to be antibody-tested. If they are antibody-positive and having safe sex with someone who is antibody-positive, both partners are probably not transmitting HIV. If the individual is antibody-negative and is planning to have safe sex with someone who is antibody-negative, then, again, both partners are probably not transmitting. Most funds for education and the greatest support are needed for those situations where one individual is antibody-positive and the other individual is antibody-negative, which can become tragedies. I believe it morally unconscionable and medically foolish for two individuals in high-risk groups to enter into a sexual relationship in which safe sex cannot be practiced 100 percent of the time and in which one or both partners do not know their antibody status.

Even persons not falling into one of the groups described above probably need this information. If they are worried about being infected with HIV, the antibody test will relieve their anxiety and they can get on with their lives. If in fact they have been infected, they can work with their health care practitioners to maintain their immune system at an optimal level. This would include exercise, diet, reduction of stress, elimination of recreational drugs, among other precautions.

Finally, this group of individuals—those that are antibody-positive and are doing all they can to ensure their survival—should also be encouraged to pay close attention to experimental drug programs that will be used in the near future to try to eliminate viral infection in AIDS, ARC, and asymptomatic individuals.

What are the symptoms associated with ARC? Please briefly explain each medical syndrome or symptom that you mention.

Briefly stated, ARC is any medical condition in an HIV antibody-positive individual that does not meet the definition of AIDS, such as KS or *Pneumocystis* pneumonia, but results from a consequence of immunosuppression. Twenty-five percent of the individuals infected with HIV develop persistent and/or recurrent lymphadenopathy at two or more sites outside the groin area (extrainguinal) for six months or longer. These people are classified as having ARC. Swollen nodes in the groin area are common in most men. Thus, a swollen node in the neck and a swollen node in the armpit for six months or more in an individual who is antibody-positive would almost certainly be classified as ARC by most authorities. Indeed, many authorities would classify this as ARC if the individual is in a high-risk group, even if his antibody status is not known.

The same now will be true of all the other conditions I mentioned. Some authorities do not want to call it ARC unless it is in a high-risk individual. Some professionals would want to see a positive antibody test result to help confirm their clinical impression that the patient in fact is suffering from ARC. Some of the other conditions that have been lumped into this group are severe, persistent, and recurrent fatigue; severe, persistent, and recurrent diarrhea or gastrointestinal problems; severe, persistent, and recurrent yeast infections of the mouth (remember that severe yeast infections of the esophagus meet the CDC criteria of AIDS); unexplained weight loss of ten pounds or more within a two-month period; unexplained and recurrent night sweats. Usually I would rather see that the patient is having sweating over the entire body rather than in localized areas. Many people normally experience some perspiration at night that is not associated with any infectious disease and is not clinically significant and does not make for a diagnosis of ARC.

A variety of cutaneous infections, including shingles, herpes zoster, persistent herpes simplex infections, cold sores, persistent wart infections, and numerous and persistent lesions of molloscum contagiosum, indicate some degree of immunosuppression. Bacterial infections, such as folliculitis and impetigo, have also been classified as ARC by some authorities, as has severe seborrheic dermatitis, which is dandruff of the scalp, central chest, and groin, and flares of acne on the face, chest, and back, and flares of psoriasis, which is an inherited, epidermal disease. Bizarre neurological problems are now being seen, and for lack of a better classification, they too are being called ARC. This includes unusual neuropathies, unusual paresis, episodes typical of presenile dementia, confusional states, and aberrant behavioral states. A viral encephalopathy has also been seen, but it is not clear whether this is due to infection with HIV, infection with some other agent such as CMV or Epstein-Barr virus, or perhaps even an aberrant antibody response. Antibodies to Epstein-Barr virus, which occur in mononucleosis, can cross-react, which means they indiscriminately attack myelin in nerve sheaths. Thus, in some cases, we may have a situation where the virus itself is not causing the neurological damage, but that antibodies to these viral agents may be attacking antigens that are present on nerve sheaths causing the neuropathy that is being seen clinically. Clearly, much more work needs to be done on this.

What else makes up ARC? Some people have included recurrent or persistent parasitosis, such as amoeba and giardia, arguing that the amoebas recur *not* because the individual has been reinfected or because of a treatment failure, but because the individual is immunosuppressed and treatment is not capable of eliminating the parasite from the intestine. It is probably true. Deposition of immune complexes in the kidney resulting in glomerulonephritis has also been seen and would probably be classified as ARC, and a form of ulcerative colitis, which is probably related to CMV infection of the colon and small intestine, has also been noted and has been classified as ARC.

Can't someone have lymphadenopathy that has no relationship to AIDS?

Yes, but such infections are indeed very rare. In most adults who have swollen lymph nodes in the neck or armpit, those nodes will subside within six months unless they represent some underlying disease such as persistent Epstein-Barr virus infection, persistent CMV infection, or HIV infection. Certain lymphomas, such as Hodgkin's disease, will also produce swollen nodes that in biopsy will reveal the malignancy. I have seen one or two patients out of maybe two or three thousand in the last five years who have had swollen nodes for six months or longer in whom there was no evidence of infection with HIV or any other viral infection. This may represent individuals who have lymph nodes larger than those of the average man and these nodes are palpable but do not represent disease.

With AIDS, I believe that a person's body recognizes the infection and starts trying to make antibodies to fight off the infection and that is why the lymph nodes in the neck and armpits swell up. When the lymph nodes go away, that is not necessarily a good sign. The lymph nodes may not be going away because the individual has successfully fought off the infection. The lymph nodes may be going away because his immune system is just totally collapsing and a few months later he will come down with pneumocystis or KS. And there is some evidence to suggest that that is correct.

> Some of my patients feel very hopeless and anxious about the future, particularly those who have ARC symptoms. What are some good ways of presenting or interpreting their medical picture?

The anxiety clearly comes from the fact that they are in limbo: they don't know if they're going to recover or progress on to AIDS, or if they are going to continue to have their current symptoms. Unhappily, we don't have the answer. We don't know what percentage of ARC patients progresses on to AIDS, what percent totally recovers, and what percentage continues to have one or many of the conditions that we've previously discussed as ARC.

Probably it is better just to reassure the patient generally that most patients with ARC are not progressing onto AIDS and focus the patient's attention on recovering from the particular ailment that has brought him to the physician at that time. If he's having fatigue, for example, work on ways of treating the fatigue. If the patient's having recurrent bowel problems, work on those, rather than focusing the patient on the uncertainty of his future. Discussing their anxiety with a therapist has been of great value to many patients, and small therapy groups of patients suffering from similar conditions have been utilized with great benefit to large numbers of patients in getting them through the anxiety of realizing they've been infected with HIV.

> Are there any other questions that people regularly ask you that merit attention?

Although there are not any specific questions that have not been addressed, I think it's important to keep focusing patients on the fact that most people infected with this agent continue to survive and not have any symptoms. And a couple of specific examples are often useful; for example, one of my patients was in his forties and his lover was in his twenties when, in 1983, the lover developed pneumocystis and died. We checked this man's helper/suppressor ratio. It was not at the normal ratio of 2 to 1. It was not down to one-tenth of normal at .2 to 1; it was not down at one-twentieth of normal at .1 to 1. Indeed, it was 0.05 to 1. He had *eight* circulating helper T-cells in his blood sample. Since 1983, he has continued to have helper T-cells in this ratio. He is alive, he is well, he has no symptoms, he has not developed AIDS or ARC. So because a person is infected with HIV does not mean that he is going to get sick. A person whose helper T-cells are totally wiped out is not necessarily going to get sick. Clearly, you cannot get AIDS unless you've been infected with HIV and it has knocked out your helper T-cells, but depletion of helper T-cells alone is not a prognostic sign that disease is going to develop.

Specific stories like that seem useful in reassuring patients that being infected with this agent does not necessarily mean a fatal outcome.

4

Neuropsychiatric Syndromes in AIDS and AIDS-Related Illnesses

DEAN L. WOLCOTT

Our knowledge is still incomplete about diseases of the central nervous system (CNS) in patients with AIDS and ARC as they contribute to the organic mental disorders common in these patient populations. The clinical implications of this developing body of knowledge for mental health professionals will be emphasized in this review. Medical and psychosocial aspects of AIDS and ARC have been reviewed elsewhere in this volume and other publications and are beyond the scope of this chapter. Adequate understanding of CNS disease states and organic mental disorders in AIDS and ARC depends on familiarity with the medical and psychosocial aspects of this epidemic. The term *neuropsychiatric syndromes* will be used to include both CNS disease states and organic mental disorders.

Neurological Disease States in AIDS and ARC

Disease of the CNS is extraordinarily common in patients with AIDS and ARC. Clinical studies of AIDS patients indicate that approximately 40 percent develop a clinical neurological syndrome during life (Snider et al. 1983, Levy, Bredesen, Rosenblum 1985). Autopsy studies indicate that at least 70 percent of AIDS patients have CNS disease at death (Levy, Bredesen, Rosenblum 1985, Reichert et al. 1983, Welch et al. 1984, Nielsen et al. 1984). Furthermore, about 10 percent of individuals who eventually develop AIDS or ARC develop a neurological syndrome as the first manifestation of their illness, as much as twelve months before developing other clinical signs of AIDS or ARC (Levy, Bredesen, Rosenblum 1985). Aseptic meningitis and herpes zoster radiculitis are the most common presenting neurological syndromes heralding eventual AIDS and ARC development.

Although a detailed knowledge of the neurological syndromes seen in AIDS and ARC is not essential for practicing mental health professionals, it is important that those treating AIDS and ARC patients know that neurological disease processes may affect all levels of the nervous system, may present subtly with gradual clinical progression, and may mimic functional psychiatric disease (e.g., conversion disorders). The neurological syndromes associated with AIDS and ARC are truly protean. (See table 4.1.)

CNS Disease in AIDS and ARC

In a review of the distribution of CNS disease processes in 315 AIDS and ARC patients with known CNS disease, Robert Levy and others (1985) show that potentially effective treatments exist for more than 60 percent of the CNS disease processes in AIDS and ARC patients, with the treatments used for specific diseases. CNS infections account for about 80 percent of all CNS disease processes in AIDS and ARC patients, with 10 percent developing CNS neoplasms, 8 percent unknown, and 3 percent cerebrovascular accidents. The specific CNS disease processes in AIDS and ARC will be discussed in more detail. It must be emphasized, however, that the treatment of CNS infections must usually be prolonged because of the individual's impaired immunity. The treatments are often toxic; the CNS infections often relapse if treatment is discontinued; and development of any of these CNS processes is prognostically ominous at the current time.

Nonviral CNS Infections

Nonviral CNS infections comprise about 50 percent of all CNS disease processes in AIDS and ARC patients. *Toxoplasma gondii* infections occur in about 32 percent of patients with CNS disease, and *Cryptococcus neoformans* infections occur in 13 percent. Other infections are much less common in this group.

From the clinical standpoint, patients with CNS *Toxoplasma gondii* infections may become lethargic or confused several days or more before developing focal neurological deficits or a diminished level of consciousness suggesting the diagnosis. About 15 percent of patients with toxoplasma infections develop seizures. Head CT scans typically show one or more cerebral ring-enhancing lesions, and magnetic resonance imaging scans may be positive when CT scans are negative. Cere-

Table 4.1. Neurological Disease States and Clinical Manifestations in Patients with AIDS and ARC

	Disease Process	Clinical Manifestations
Cerebrum	Acute meningitis Acute encephalitis Acute meningoencephalitis Cerebrovascular accident	Headache, nausea, vomiting, fever, lethargy, delirium, meningeal irritation, expressive language dysfunction, focal neurological deficits, seizures
	Mass lesions (infections, neoplasms)	Seizures, hydrocephalus, movement disorders, focal neurological deficits, increased intracranial pressure
	Chronic meningitis Chronic meningo-encephalitis Chronic encephalitis	As above, plus cortical atrophy, dementia, organic affective and personality syndromes
Brainstem	Meningitis Infections Neoplasms	Long tract dysfunction (motor, sensory), impaired respiratory and cardiovascular regulation
Cerebellum	Infections, neoplasms	Gait disorders, incoordination
Spinal Cord	Posterolateral column Lateral column (ALS) Viral myelitis	Sensation impairment, motor (flaccid, spastic) incontinence
Neuropathies, Myopathy	Cranial and peripheral	Sensory and motor dysfunction
	mononeuropathies and neuropathies, radiculitis myopathy, polymyositis	(e.g., distal symmetrical), Bell's palsy, dermatomal pain, muscle pain, tenderness, and wasting

brospinal fluid (CSF) findings may include increased concentrations of protein, with glucose concentrations and numbers of white blood cells variable. About 50 percent of toxoplasma lesions involve the basal ganglia. Although treatment with pyrimethamine and sulfadiazine is used, the mortality rate with CNS toxoplasma infections in this population is about 70 percent, with 30 percent of those who originally respond to treatment relapsing after treatment is stopped (Levy, Bredesen, Rosenblum 1985).

CNS infections with *Cryptococcus neoformans* usually present with headache, confusion, and/or seizures. Anatomically, these infections are usually a granulomatous meningitis, with granulomas or cysts developing in the cerebral hemispheres. Head CT scans may be normal, show cerebral atrophy, or hydrocephalus. CSF studies may be normal, although positive India ink preparations or CSF cryptococcal antigen titers may make the diagnosis. Although treatable with amphotericin B and 5-fluorocytosine, CNS *Cryptococcus neoformans* infections in AIDS and ARC patients often recur after treatment is stopped and have a 50 percent mortality rate (Levy, Bredesen, Rosenblum 1985).

Viral Infections Causing CNS Syndromes

Viral infections account for about 30 percent of CNS disease processes in AIDS and ARC patients. Although herpes simplex encephalitis, PML, and other viral infections have been reported, it is safe to infer that the majority of viral CNS disease processes are caused by CNS infection with HIV itself. The syndromes associated with CNS HIV infections include acute and chronic encephalitis, acute and chronic meningitis, peripheral neuropathy, and chronic myelopathy.

The evidence is now very strong that HIV is neurotropic and may infect the CNS within a very short interval after the first systemic infection with the virus (Carne et al. 1985, Goldwater et al. 1985, Black 1985). CNS HIV infection also may be chronic and appears to be the major cause of the subacute encephalitis/dementia syndrome (Ho et al. 1985). The common clinical neuropsychiatric syndromes associated with CNS HIV infection will be briefly described.

Cooper et al. (1985) have previously documented that acute systemic HIV infection with first development of HIV antibodies is often associated with an acute mononucleosislike syndrome with fever, myalgias, headache, and malaise. A rapidly fatal illness in a promiscuous, previously healthy homosexual man was described by Goldwater et al. (1985). He had clinical evidence of acute meningoencephalitis during life, and autopsy revealed gross evidence of temporal lobe, hippocampal, and hypothalamic involvement, with microscopic findings strongly suggestive of acute HIV infection. He did not have evidence of impaired immunity during life and did not meet the criteria for the diagnosis of AIDS.

Carne et al. (1985) have recently reported three patients with an acute viral encephalitis associated with probable acute HIV infection as manifested by antibody seroconversion (appearance of HIV antibodies in serum). All three had neurological symptoms and evidence of delirium with personality and affective changes. Two had generalized EEG abnormalities and also onset of generalized seizures. All three recovered after a short illness course, though one continued to have altered personality.

Ho et al. (1985) have confirmed the role of HIV infection in many cases of acute and chronic meningitis, myelopathy, and neuropathy in AIDS and ARC patients. They also isolated HIV from CNS specimens of ten/sixteen AIDS patients with the subacute encephalitis/dementia syndrome, providing further evidence that this syndrome is often, if not always, secondary to HIV infection (also Snider et al. 1983, Shaw et al. 1985, Resnick et al. 1985, Levy, Shimabukuro et al. 1985). Clinically, patients with this syndrome typically have a chronic progressive course of intellectual, social, and psychological deterioration. (See next chapter.) Late manifestations include advanced dementia with confusion, seizures, language disorders including mutism, loss of bladder and bowel control, gait disturbances and inability to walk, and coma (Holland, Tross 1985). Neurological symptoms at presentation may include confusion, fever, focal neurological signs, seizures, and frontal release signs. Head CT scans are often normal in the early stages, but usually later show generalized cortical atrophy and ventricular enlargement. CSF studies are usually abnormal but not always, with mild increased CSF protein and +/− decreased glucose concentrations. EEG studies usually find diffuse generalized slowing. Anatomic studies post mortem often indicate greatest involvement of the hypothalamus and brainstem, with microscopic findings of microglial nodules in the gray matter (Snider et al. 1983, Levy, Bredesen, Rosenblum 1985).

Recent evidence also indicates that HIV infection is frequently the cause of acute and chronic aseptic meningitis in AIDS and ARC patients (Levy, Bredesen, Rosenblum 1985, Ho et al. 1985). This syndrome almost always occurs in patients with ARC, whereas the subacute encephalitis syndrome almost always occurs in AIDS patients. This syndrome may present with headache, fever, meningeal signs, cranial neuropathy (V, VII, VIII), and/or long tract signs. Head CT scans are usually negative, and by definition CSF demonstrates pleiocytosis, with usually increased protein and decreased CSF glucose levels. Aseptic meningitis is usually self-limited, but may recur. Treatment is symptomatic.

Thus, clinical and autopsy evidence strongly indicates that active

HIV infections of the brain and spinal chord are major contributors to the neurological syndromes seen in AIDS and ARC patients. HIV infections may coexist with other infectious and neoplastic processes causing neurological morbidity in AIDS (Ho et al. 1985).

CNS Neoplastic Processes

CNS neoplasms are a less frequent cause of CNS disease in AIDS and ARC patients. B-cell lymphomas, which may be primary to the CNS or associated with systemic lymphoma, and KS have been reported (Levy, Bredesen, Rosenblum 1985, Loewenstein, Rubinow forthcoming). Levine has reported that 30 percent of homosexual males with B-cell lymphoma had neurological symptoms at the time of tumor diagnosis, and an additional 14 percent developed CNS symptoms during the course of treatment, an unusually high incidence of CNS involvement (Levine et al. 1985). Patients with CNS KS may have symptomatic CNS bleeding (Levy, Bredesen, Rosenblum 1985, Loewenstein, Rubinow forthcoming).

Cerebrovascular Disorders

A small percentage of CNS disorders in AIDS and ARC patients are related to CNS bleeding from ITP, cerebrovascular emboli from nonbacterial endocarditis, and possibly cerebral arteritis (Snider et al. 1983, Levy, Bredesen, Rosenblum 1985).

Organic Mental Disorders

Organic mental disorders (OMD) are very common in patients with AIDS and ARC (Holland, Tross 1985, Wolcott, Fawzy, Pasnau 1985, Ho et al. 1985, Loewenstein, Rubinow forthcoming). The major acute OMD seen in this population is delirium. The most common chronic OMD is dementia, with organic affective syndromes and organic personality syndromes occurring. Although exact figures on the incidence and prevalence of OMD in AIDS and ARC patients are not available, reasonable clinical estimates suggest that 40–70 percent of AIDS and ARC patients develop an OMD during the course of their illness (Wolcott, Fawzy, Pasnau 1985, Loewenstein, Rubinow forthcoming, Perry, Tross 1984). The prevalence of OMD in AIDS patients seems to increase with duration of illness and is more common in patients with opportunistic infections than in patients whose only basis for the diagnosis of AIDS is KS.

Acute OMD

Clinically, delirium is the predominant acute OMD in this patient population. The official diagnostic criteria for delirium are described in the *Diagnostic and Statistical Manual of Mental Disorders* (American Psychiatric Association 1980). (See next chapter.) Although many of the clinical features of delirium and dementia are the same, the cardinal distinguishing clinical characteristic of delirium is an altered (and/or fluctuating) level of consciousness. Although the official diagnostic criteria are clinically useful, it is important to recognize that delirium is a dynamic process of generalized cognitive dysfunction based on generalized dysfunction of cortical and subcortical anatomic structures. Thus, delirium may range in severity from being subtle and requiring astute clinical diagnosis to severe obtundation obvious to even non–mental health professionals. Minor changes are often present in delirious patients before florid cognitive dysfunction develops.

Delirium in AIDS and ARC patients is often misdiagnosed as a depression or other functional psychiatric syndrome. Typically, delirium in medically ill patients has an acute onset, is multifactorial in etiology, and resolves completely within four to seven days without neurological or cognitive sequelae. (See table 4.2.) The basis of treatment of delirium in this population can be summarized as follows: Completely evaluate the patient medically. Treat all treatable contributing medical conditions. In regard to the psychological and environment support, (1) explain to the patient and significant others about the nature of delirium, its usual course, and expected degree of reversibility; (2) provide frequent contact with a small number of individuals who are well known to the individual (significant others, medical staff); (3) provide frequent orienting cues (e.g., date, time, place, situation, reasons for procedures, soft light at night); (4) minimize all medications that depress the cerebral cortex (e.g., analgesics, sedative hypnotics); (5) try to help restore usual biorhythms (e.g., sleep cycle); (6) offer frequent, brief supportive psychotherapy sessions, and evaluate frequently for suicidal ideation and impulsivity. As for psychopharmacologic treatment, use low-dose high-potency neuroleptics when needed for treatment of severe anxiety and/or agitated and potentially dangerous behavior.

Table 4.2. Organic Mental Disorders in AIDS and ARC*

I. Delirium (contributing factors)

A. Primary CNS disease states

1. Infectious, neoplastic, cerebrovascular disease states as in the chronic organic mental disorders

2. Meningitis and meningoencephalitis—acute HIV, B-cell lymphoma, Kaposi's sarcoma; fungal, atypical mycobacterial, and possible other viral infections

3. Other—seizure disorder and posticial states, treatment side effects (e.g., chemotherapy, interferon)

B. CNS abnormalities secondary to systemic processes—sepsis, hypoxemia from respiratory compromise (e.g., *Pneumocystis carinii* pneumonia), electrolyte imbalance

C. Environmental and psychological factors—visual loss, sensory understimulation, inactivity, disrupted circadian rhythms, psychological distress, social isolation, sleep loss

II. Chronic Organic Mental Disorders

A. Dementia (process/agents)

1. Diffuse subacute encephalitis—HIV, probably CMV, and possible other

2. Other progressive viral encephalitic syndromes—herpes simplex virus, progressive multifocal leukoencephalopathy, varicella-zoster virus

3. Cerebral mass lesions— *Toxoplasma gondii, Cryptococcus neoformans, Candida albicans,* polymicrobial, possible other infections; B-cell lymphoma, Kaposi's sarcoma

4. Cerebrovascular accident—cerebral hemorrhage, nonbacterial thrombotic endocarditis, cerebral arteritis

5. Possible butritional deficiency

B. Organic affective syndrome and organic personality syndrome-subacute encephalitis (HIV), and possibly others

---

*Adapted from Wolcott, Fawzy, Pasnau 1985.

Readers interested in more detailed discussions of the diagnosis and management of delirium in general and in AIDS and ARC patients are referred to several reviews (Holland, Tross 1985, Wolcott, Fawzy, Pasnau 1985, Loewenstein, Rubinow forthcoming, Lipowski 1985). The development of delirium is a psychiatric and usually medical emergency in AIDS and ARC patients, and all such patients should be hospitalized and receive careful general medical, neurological, and psychiatric care.

Chronic OMD

The official diagnostic criteria for dementia are described in the *DSM* (American Psychiatric Association 1980). (See next chapter.) Characteristic late clinical features of dementia in AIDS and ARC patients have been described in the section on subacute encephalitis. The high frequency and severity of dementia in AIDS and ARC patients represent one of the greatest challenges the health care delivery system faces in responding to the AIDS epidemic in the United States. Currently, no effective treatment is known against HIV, and eradication of the organism from the CNS will prove difficult, if not impossible, in the near future (Black 1985). Dementia associated with other CNS infections or neoplasms may respond to effective medical treatment of the underlying CNS disease process.

Dementia associated with HIV may have a subtle onset, which may easily be mistaken for a functional psychiatric syndrome. I have seen many AIDS patients with the subacute encephalitis/dementia syndrome that presented as apparently classical functional psychiatric syndromes including generalized anxiety disorders, panic attacks, endogenous depressive episodes, acute paranoid psychoses, bipolar episodes, and schizophreniform psychoses. My clinical observation is substantiated by others (Dilley, Macks 1986). Table 4.2 contains information about the frequent contributing factors to dementia in AIDS and ARC patients. Treatment is based on the same principles as treatment of delirium, summarized above. Because of the severity of personal deterioration common in dementia in AIDS patients, adequate management requires a multidisciplinary team that carefully plans a comprehensive patient management program. It includes evaluation of the patient's need for financial support, activities of daily living and self-care assistance, legal protection according to the patient's condition, and ability and desire to participate in medical treatment decisions. There is increasing recognition of clinical differences between dementia primarily involving cerebral cortical structures and dementia arising from dysfunction of subcortical structures (Cummings, Benson 1983). Subcortical dementia may be the most common form of dementia in individuals infected with HIV, and it can affect memory, language, motor, and integrative functions (Holland, Tross 1985).

The highly variable clinical course of dementia associated with CNS HIV infection in AIDS causes special problems in diagnosis and management. Some patients will have a gradually deteriorating course over months before becoming seriously impaired. Others will have a very dramatic onset, suggestive of acute HIV encephalitis, which then progresses to profound dementia in a few days to weeks. This clinical observation leads to difficulties in distinguishing delirium and dementia in some AIDS patients. Whereas in other patient populations delirium typically resolves without sequelae, in AIDS patients it may rapidly progress to dementia.

Organic affective syndromes and organic personality syndromes also occur in AIDS patients. Although the evidence about frequency and etiology of these syndromes in AIDS patients is not in, in most cases these syndromes are associated with CNS HIV infection.

Subclinical Cognitive Impairment

Holland and Tross (1985) have reported that about 80 percent of AIDS patients without known neurological complications at the onset of their study showed cognitive impairment in one or more of seven areas tested that involved memory, integrative, and language function. Loewenstein and Rubinow (forthcoming) have quoted from an unpublished NIH study conducted by Joffe et al. of neuropsychological function in thirteen male homosexual AIDS patients free of known CNS or systemic complications of their disease. When compared to a sample of healthy homosexual males, matched in age and education, the AIDS patients had significantly lower scores on full-scale IQ and verbal IQ tests, several WAIS subtests, the Halstead Category Test, and the Trailmaking B test. They concluded that the AIDS patients had diffuse cerebral dysfunction and particularly dominant hemisphere and language impairment.

Role of Mental Health Professionals in the Diagnosis and Management of Neuropsychiatric Syndromes

The high incidence of neurological disease processes in individuals with HIV infection, the high incidence and severity of OMD in AIDS and ARC patients, the frequency with which neurological disease processes may initially present with psychiatric symptoms, and the importance to the patient of accurate and early diagnosis of a neuropsychiatric syndrome when present—all mean that mental health professionals treating AIDS and ARC patients have a significant clinical responsibility to recognize neuropsychiatric syndromes in these individuals. Because OMD in AIDS and ARC patients may present as classical functional psychiatric syndromes, any psychiatric syndrome in these patients should be considered an OMD until proven otherwise. An OMD caused by a primary CNS disease process in AIDS and ARC patients may be present for weeks or months before the development of other neurological symptoms or signs of CNS disease. A CNS disease may be present even if all neurodiagnostic tests are normal or nondiagnostic. Common CNS disease states in AIDS and ARC patients that may present with psychiatric symptoms include: subacute encephalitis/dementia, atypical aseptic meningitis, primary CNS lymphoma, and *Toxoplasma gondii* infections. Some CNS disease states that cause OMD in these patients are medically treatable.

Careful attention to changes in psychological status and social function; well-developed skills in the examination of the mental status of patients to detect cognitive impairment; the knowledge and skill to diagnose accurately clinical organic mental disorders in patients; referral to neurological specialists when a neurological disorder is detected or suspected; and skill in the management of delirium and dementia are all essential to optimal fulfillment of mental health professionals' responsibility to their AIDS and ARC patients. Any program that provides psychiatric, psychological, and/or social services to AIDS and ARC patients has an important responsibility to ensure that all clinical staff members have enough knowledge of neuropsychiatric syndromes in AIDS and ARC at least to perform an accurate screening function in the clinical care of these individuals. Adequate care of neuropsychiatric syndromes in AIDS and ARC patients often requires the efforts of a multidisciplinary team of neurologists, neuropsychologists, clinical psychopharmacologists, and psychotherapists.

References

American Psychiatric Association. 1980. *Diagnostic and statistical manual of mental disorders*. 3d ed. Washington, D.C.: American Psychiatric Association Press.

Black, P. H. 1985. HTLV-III, AIDS, and the brain. *N Engl J Med* 313: 1538–40.

Carne, C. A., R. S. Tedder, A. Smith, et al. 1985. Acute encephalopathy coincident with seroconversion for anti-HTLV-III. *Lancet* 2 : 1206–8.

Cooper, D. A., J. Gold, P. Maclean, et al. 1985. Acute AIDS retrovirus infection: Definition of a clinical illness associated with seroconversion. *Lancet* 1 : 537–40.

Cummings, J. L., and D. F. Benson. 1983. *Dementia: A clinical approach.* Boston: Butterworths.

DeVita, V. T., Jr., S. Hellman, and S. A. Rosenberg, eds. 1985. *AIDS: Etiology, diagnosis, treatment, and prevention.* Philadelphia: J. B. Lippincott.

Dilley, J., and J. Macks. 1986. Secondary depression in AIDS. Data presented at International Conference on AIDS, June 23. Paris, France.

Fauci, A. S., H. Masur, E. P. Gelmann, et al. 1985. The acquired immunodeficiency syndrome: An update. *Ann Int Med* 102 : 800–13.

Forstein, M. 1984. The psychosocial impact of the acquired immunodeficiency syndrome. *Ann Int Med* 1103 : 765–67.

Goldwater, P. N., B. J. L. Synek, T. D. Koelmeyer, P. J. Scott. 1985. Structures resembling scrapie-associated fibrils in AIDS encephalopathy. *Lancet* 2 : 447–48.

Ho, D. D., T. R. Rota, R. T. Schooley, et al. 1985. Isolation of HTLV-III from cerebrospinal fluid and neural tissues of patients with neurologic syndromes related to the acquired immunodeficiency syndrome. *N Engl J Med* 313 : 1493–97.

Holland, J. C., and S. Tross. 1985. Psychosocial and neuropsychiatric sequelae of the acquired immunodeficiency syndrome and related disorders. *Ann Int Med* 103 : 760–64.

Levine, A. M., S. G. Parkash, P. R. Meyer, et al. 1985. Retrovirus and malignant lymphoma in homosexual men. *JAMA* 254 : 1921–25.

Levy, J. A., J. Shimabukuro, H. Hollander, et al. 1985. Isolation of AIDS-associated retroviruses from cerebrospinal fluid and brain of patients with neurological symptoms. *Lancet* 2 : 586–88.

Levy, R. M., D. E. Bredesen, M. L. Rosenblum. 1985. Neurological manifestations of the acquired immunodeficiency syndrome (AIDS): Experience at UCSF and review of the literature. *J Neurosurg* 62 : 475–95.

Lipowski, Z. J. 1985. Delirium (acute Confusional State). In *Handbook of clinical neurology. Neurobehavioral disorders*, ed. J. A. M. Fredericks. Vol. 2. New York: Elsevier, pp. 523–59.

Loewenstein, R. J., D. R. Rubinow. Forthcoming. Psychiatric aspects of AIDS: The organic mental syndromes. In *Viruses, Immunity, and Mental Diseases*, ed. M. T. Kurstak and Z. J. Lipowski. New York: Plenum.

Morin, S. F., K. A. Charles, and A. K. Malyon. 1984. The psychological impact of AIDS on gay men. *Am Psychologist* 39:1288–93.

Nichols, S. E. 1985. Psychosocial reactions of persons with the acquired immunodeficiency syndrome. *Ann Int Med* 103:765–67.

Nielsen, S., C. K. Petito, C. D. Urmacher, et al. 1984. Subacute encephalitis in acquired immune deficiency syndrome: A postmortem study. *Am J Clin Pathol* 82:678–82.

Perry, S. W., and S. Tross. 1984. Psychiatric problems of AIDS inpatients at the New York Hospital: Preliminary report. *Pub Hlth Rep* 99:200–205.

Petito, C. K., B. A. Navia, E. S. Cho, et al. 1985. Vacuolar myelopathy pathologically resembling subacute combined degeneration in patients with the acquired immunodeficiency syndrome. *N Engl J Med* 312:874–79.

Resnick, L., F. DiMarzo-Veronese, J. Schupbach, et al. 1985. Intra-blood-brain-barrier synthesis of HTLV-III-specific IgG in patients with neurologic symptoms associated with AIDS or AIDS-related complex. *N Engl J Med* 313:1498–1504.

Shaw, G. M., M. E. Harper, B. H. Hahn, et al. 1985. HTLV-III infection in brains of children and adults with AIDS encephalopathy. *Science* 227:177–82.

5

The Role of Psychiatry: Evaluation and Treatment of the Altered Mental Status in Persons with AIDS

SAMUEL TUCKER

The psychiatric management of AIDS-related psychosis and organic deterioration as an emergent discipline has been only gradually recognized. Although published data about AIDS-related psychiatric problems has been minimal, I fear that a great deal more psychiatric problems will emerge as the epidemic continues. The majority of my information comes from anecdotal case reports in the psychiatric literature, from other colleagues, and from personal experience (Holland, Tross 1985, Hoffman 1984, Kermani, Drab, Alpert 1984, Loewenstein, Scharfstein 1983–84).

AIDS is frequently complicated by central nervous system dysfunctions. (See preceding chapter.) Dementia in the absence of opportunistic infections is also being recognized as a primary presentation of AIDS. It is now strongly asserted that HIV is neurotropic—that is, it attacks the neurons—and it is the probable cause for these progressive dementing processes (Shaw et al. 1985). One report showed that only 19 of the 110 patients were without neurological changes at autopsy (Jordan et al. 1985). I also have anecdotal reports from colleagues that up to 50 to 70 percent of the patients that they have seen in consultation demonstrated certain aspects of dementia.

When a psychiatric consultation is requested on AIDS patients because of mental status changes, one is confronted with the need to assess rapidly whether the cause of the process is potentially treatable. Delineating an etiology is imperative in order to expedite appropriate medical treatment. Opportunistic infections and their concomitant high fevers, polypharmacy, or specific agents such as amphotericin B, which is used for cryptococcosis and other fungal infections, may all foster altered mental status. The psychiatric consultant must be prepared to assess and differentiate deliriums from depression or dementia, which have overlapping symptoms.

Delirious patients may be differentiated by several specific features. A delirium is usually of rapid onset, occurring over some hours to days. Delirious patients tend to show increased psychomotor activity, such as agitated pacing or rocking. Their sleep–wakefulness pattern may also be altered, with more activity at night. Psychotic sensory–perceptual disturbances, including visual, auditory, and somatic hallucinations and persecutory delusions are not uncommon in these people. A clouded sensorium, making any cognitive testing impossible, is also a hallmark of a delirious state. In other words, the patients are grossly disoriented, not knowing where they are or what is happening to them.

Many AIDS patients are presenting with some of the aspects of these symptoms. Deliriums, as a rule, tend to have a traceable and often a treatable etiology. Examples of this are, perhaps, the severe bitemporal headaches of incipient cryptococcal meningitis, or drug toxicity from one or several combined medications that may foster a delirium state.

If a treatable delirium or focal lesion is ruled out, the psychiatric consultant must next differentiate between a functional depression and dementia as the reason for the mental status changes. One-third to one-fifth of all hospitalized medically ill patients manifest some form of depressive symptomatology (Derogatis et al. 1983). The diagnosis of major depression in medically ill patients is clouded because many of the symptoms of depression may also result from their medical illness. Fatigue, weight loss, difficulty in sleeping, and anorexia are all symptoms held in common by AIDS and depression.

To differentiate between depression and a medical etiology, one should emphasize cognitive and affective symptoms while minimizing their somatic concerns (Cavanaugh 1983). Certain aspects of the Beck Depression and Hopelessness Scale are helpful in making this diagnosis. These include presence of low self-esteem, feeling like a failure, loss of interest in other people and relationships, feeling as if being punished for something, recurrent suicidal ideation, difficulty carrying through in making decisions and, also, frequent crying spells. A history of major depression, previous psychiatric treatment, particularly with medication, or suicide attempts in the past also give clues as to whether or not this is a functional depression as opposed to dementia.

Nevertheless, an unexplained onset of depression in AIDS patients who had formerly been coping adequately with their disease may herald the onset of a central nervous system process other than just a functional depression. Case reports in the psychiatric and medical literature describe a dementing process attributable to AIDS. Dementing illnesses are usually of an insidious onset; they occur over a long period of time. And they are marked by a clear sensorium in the presence of measurable cognitive deficits. Such deficits include the inability to retain new information, confusion, disorientation, and short- and long-term memory deficits. These parameters are also true for the organicity that is beginning to be seen in AIDS patients.

The case reports describe patients who are confused, with a loss of interest in personal appearance and hygiene, and displaying inappropriate behaviors in public. The spectrum of presentation ranges from a pathetic, passive cooperation—an almost lobotomized attitude—and total unconcern about the situation to temper tantrums, inappropriate disrobing, decreased frustration tolerance, affective lability, anxiety, paranoia, suspiciousness, hostility, and delusional and frankly psychotic thought processes. On examination, most show what are called "frontal release signs" in the absence of any focal neurological findings. Serial EEGs may demonstrate diffuse slowing, and CT scans may show cortical atrophy with a ventricular enlargement. Many of these patients are appearing in psychiatric hospitals without a previous AIDS diagnosis. Only serial cognitive assessments, abnormal EEGs, and CT scans permit the eventual diagnosis of a dementing process resulting from AIDS.

What possible treatments and interventions do we have? They do not raise great expectations. Treatment of delirium primarily entails addressing the underlying etiology. As was mentioned, illnesses such as infectious agents may be treated, which allows the patient to return to the usual level of adaptive functioning. Polypharmacy, causing altered mental status, or the presence of street drugs or much alcohol must also be eliminated in order for the client to clear his sensorium. In the functionally psychotic, severely agitated, or deliriously demented patient, neuroleptic medication may be necessary. High-potency, low-anticholinergic medications such as haloperidol or thiothixene at *minimal* doses are favored to clear these states for several reasons. They reduce agitation and eliminate psychotic ideation without too much sedation or without problems causing orthostatic hypotension, and they do not significantly lower the seizure threshold. Avoiding medication with anticholinergic activity—chlorpromazine and thioridazine are just two—is preferred because the patient has a central nervous system dysfunction and may be taking other medications. Anticholinergic activity can exacerbate the disorientation, causing memory difficulties and even producing a toxic psychosis. Moreover, anticholinergic activity dries the secretions of the oral and pharyngeal membranes, which are an inhibiting mechanism in the growth of opportunistic infections like thrush or *Candida*. Benzodiazepines, another class of medications, which includes diazepam, should be avoided for a delirious patient, as they tend to increase confusion and agitation by depressing higher cortical function.

The treatment of depression also entails the use of the least anticholinergic medications. The drugs most commonly used are alprazolam and trazedone. Reports indicate that trazedone causes an often reversible process called priapism, and therefore alprazolam is usually the drug of choice. If the patient is severely ill and *extremely* depressed, when rapid mobilization is needed, you can use a stimulant such as methylphenipate, being aware that insomnia, agitation, and tachycardia are troublesome side effects of such stimulants and also of other stimulants, such as amphetamines.

This discussion about medication should not overshadow the basic importance of various therapy techniques, such as supportive, insight, cognitive, and behavioral models, in order to help patients cope with the extremely difficult process they are undergoing, and also to help dementing patients who still have sufficient cognitive capabilities to understand what is happening to them.

Successful treatment of AIDS dementia entails much more than just medications for all involved. One needs to turn to a parallel literature to find a successful model for the management of the dementing patient—both in the hospital and in the community. The Alzheimer's patient, suffering from another progressive dementing illness, provides one successful model (Powell and Courtice 1985, Reisberg 1983). On an inpatient basis, a staff educated to recognize and care for people who are undergoing a dementing process should be able to contain patients' behavior. In-service programs are imperative to educate nursing staffs in management strategies for dementing patients. This is particularly important on medical wards where nurses may not be accustomed to working with patients with behavioral problems like those seen in organic diseases—especially with AIDS patients, who so often are quite young.

Management on medical wards can be enhanced by placing patients on an involuntary status if the staff feels they are gravely disabled, which means unable to provide housing, food, or shelter for themselves, or by accepting them on an inpatient basis. Involuntary status allows some hospitals to provide round-the-clock sitters to assist nurses in controlling and monitoring difficult behaviors. I am not quite sure if staffs on medical wards know what that means. In psychiatry we often have to place patients on an involuntary basis if they are suicidal, homicidal, or unable to care for themselves. If you place someone on an involuntary basis, many insurance carriers including MediCal and Medicare will then allow for the payment of continuous sitters, whose presence can greatly enhance nursing care in monitoring difficult behaviors.

On an outpatient basis, the overall strategy is simply to keep patients as functionally autonomous as is medically responsible and feasible. Early on in the AIDS dementia, depending on the level of cognitive impairment and physical stamina, patients may be allowed to go home and may function adequately with minimal assistance. Later, as the disease and the dementing process continue, patients may require closer supervision, eventually even round-the-clock care-givers. This supervision can be an overwhelming burden to lovers, family, and friends, who usually are the ones able and willing to provide this needed service. For Alzheimer's patients and, we hope, for AIDS patients, we are going to have to develop "respite programs." These must be created in order to alleviate periodically the tremendous responsibilities of the care-givers, who can place dementing or sick patients in a hospital or convalescent home for a brief circumscribed period of time.

Educational programs for care-givers about the disease, the responsibilities involved, and how to use community services are crucial. Support groups for care-givers have to be developed; and day-care programs may also have to be developed in the future. Public health and home visiting nurses will have to make regular assessments during the course of the disease. Therefore, these professionals, too, will need extensive in-service programs to learn evaluatory and management skills.

Many factors have to be considered about the personal safety of patients in the home. Considerations include: Can an individual patient dress himself, take his medication, or medications, especially those that may be toxic in combination? Can he take care of laundry, buy food, cook meals, or simply feed himself? Is he able to count money in order to be able to shop? Able to drive a car? To take a cab? Or a bus? Is he able to follow through on any given task? These questions must be assessed in an ongoing manner as the disease progresses.

Reality orientation devices must be placed in the home for the patient's environmental safety. Such devices include very large calendars and signs that define and distinguish rooms and their functions (you would be surprised how many people cannot even remember what is in a room when the door is closed). Signs over the stove that say, for example, "Turn it off," or "Is the gas turned off?" are valuable if these patients forget from moment to moment what to do and where and how to do it. A current picture of patients should be available to identify them to the police in case they wander away from home. Firearms and other weapons must be removed. Demented people are frequently paranoid and may also be suicidal. They may accidentally or purposefully hurt themselves or others. These are just a few of the practical tips that help keep someone safely at home as long as is medically feasible and responsible.

In conclusion, the goals of the interventions described are to maintain patients at their highest level of adaptive functioning and to maintain their greatest degree of autonomy, personal integrity, and independence as well as to address and treat those processes that can be treated until the time that it is possible to cure them.

References

Cavanaugh, S. 1983. Diagnosing depression in the hospitalized medically ill. *Psychosomatics* 24:809–15.

Derogatis, L. R., G. R. Morrow, J. Fetting, et al. 1983. The prevalence of psychiatric disorders among cancer patients. *JAMA* 249:751–57.

Hoffman, R. 1984. Neuropsychiatric complications of AIDS. *Psychosomatics* 25:393–400.

Holland, J. C., and S. Tross. 1985. Psychosocial and neuropsychiatric sequelae of the acquired immunodeficiency syndrome and related disorders. *Ann Int Med* 103:760–64.

Jordan, B., B. A. Navia, S. Cho, et al. 1985. Neurological complications of AIDS: An overview based on 110 autopsied patients. In *Proceedings of the international conference on AIDS*, p. 49. Atlanta, Georgia.

Kermani, E., S. Drab, M. Alpert. 1984. Organic brain syndrome in three cases of AIDS. *Comp Psychiatry* 25:294–97.

Loewenstein, R. J., and S. S. Sharfstein. 1983–84. Neuropsychiatric aspects of AIDS. *Int J Psychiatry in Medicine* 13:255–61.

Powell, L. S., and K. Courtice. 1985. *Alzheimer's disease*. Menlo Park, Calif.: Addison-Wesley.

Reisberg, B. 1983. *Guide to Alzheimer's disease*. New York: Free Press.

Shaw, G. M., M. E. Harper, B. H. Hahn, et al. 1985. HTLV-III infections in brains of children and adults with AIDS encephalopathy. *Science* 227:177–82.

6

Medicine and the Psychology of Treating the Terminally Ill

JEROME SCHOFFERMAN

Mental health issues are, of course, profoundly pertinent to patients with AIDS and to those who work with AIDS patients. Literature on physical symptom management of the terminally ill abounds and guidelines are provided for the best applications of this knowledge: the management of pain, nausea and vomiting, shortness of breath, and other problems with which physicians and nurses are most familiar. As for the psychology involved in treating the terminally ill, I know what I do, and I know what the nurses, social workers, and volunteers at Hospice do. Yet it is difficult to put this art of medicine into terms that can be helpful for professional and lay people interested in this area. A combination of literature that articulates this area of care and personal impressions of my own work will perhaps describe it best.

One mistake we have made time and time again in medicine is the reinforcement of the mind-body dichotomy, separating the person's physical problems from the psychological ones. I would like to ensure that the same mistake does not happen in reverse, that is, mental health practitioners consider the mental health aspects out of context of the physical problems. Mental health workers need to know the physical problems associated with AIDS. They need to keep up with new treatments and new means of diagnosis. Patients frequently come to us not knowing what to expect and yet we need to be able to intervene on a meaningful level. Frequently, discussion of symptoms—discussion of the illness on a physical level—is an entry point from which to help the patients on all levels. Furthermore, most AIDS patients are under the care not of mental health workers but of primary care physicians and nurses. Therefore, the mental health issues extend well beyond the usually assigned roles of the mental health practitioner.

Doubtless, many health professionals have thought, perhaps often, what it means to be given a diagnosis of AIDS. It means that the person receiving it is going to have a struggle with chronic illness for the rest of his life and has the very real possibility, if not the assurance, that he is going to lose the struggle. That person's present is immediately shattered at the time the diagnosis is made, and his future is shattered also. I will try to share what I think are some of the meanings of being given such a diagnosis in order to anticipate what different persons' reactions might be. I will discuss briefly the art of delivering bad news, something that is often neglected and something that most of us hate to do; the nature of suffering and the goal of medicine to relieve that suffering; depression in the dying patient; and lastly, some of the specific things that care-givers can do to help.

The care of the dying patient begins with the diagnosis of a potentially fatal illness. That is to say, much of what is conveyed in that first interaction, usually with a physician, may have more meaning, or more impact, and stay with the patient longer than anything else that happens to the patient along the way. That first presentation of diagnosis is therefore critical. It should *not* be left to inexperienced people who have not delivered this sort of news or who have not at least observed it being done thoughtfully. It should be done by a physician who knows the patient and has some sort of a relationship with him. I say physician because I believe that in our society physicians have a certain power. This does not mean that physicians are better or worse or any different, it is just a role that some of us have been given along the way. But if we use that role and its power properly, we can actually help our patients through the nonspecific effect of faith in the physician.

How do we deliver bad news? In Charles Garfield's book, *The Psychosocial Care of the Dying Patient* (1978)—a book that contains much helpful information—a paper by Howard Hogshead makes many useful points.

First, *keep it simple*. Often, our own anxiety is so high when we have to tell a patient he or she has a serious disease that we start to talk nonstop and faster and faster and pretty soon we confuse the patient and do not allow the patient to get in a word. Our anxiety can lead to constant talking, often using words the patient does not understand, and not giving the patient a chance to ask any questions. So keep it simple, and use words that the patient understands.

Anticipate what the diagnosis means to that patient. This will allow you to answer some questions before they are asked and show the patient that you are experienced and will be able to help. Will I have pain? Will I suffer? Will I lose my breath? Explain some of these things in an anticipatory fashion.

Don't feel you have to deliver all the news at once. A patient can absorb and retain only a certain amount of information at one time, and that varies. We all have had the experience of being told, "The doctor never told me anything," after the patient and doctor had spent an hour discussing the problem. Do not try to deliver all the news at once. Listen for clues that suggest the patient is saturated. Give the news time to sink in, before elaborating, perhaps at the next visit.

Wait for questions. The therapeutic pause is a very effective means for allowing the patient to express his feelings, be tearful or angry, or to ask any questions.

Do not argue with denial. If a patient needs to deny after a certain point, that's fine. The patient will allow more and more entry as he gains confidence in us and feels we are being honest. Elisabeth Kubler-Ross has said that the first three times you say something to a patient might be for the patient, but the fourth time you are doing it for yourself. So, do not be overly confrontive. Allow a certain amount of denial.

I find it useful to *ask some questions of the patient.* Ask the patient to repeat to you what has been said. See that it is understood.

Leave some hope, but do not lie. You can always present the cup as being 10 percent full or 90 percent empty. Miracles happen. All of us have seen patients go into remission. So, leave some hope.

Finally, *always tell the truth,* the whole truth, and nothing but the truth. The truth sets you free. I really believe that if you tell a little lie, even in "the best interests of the patient," if you do not write down that lie on your chart, the next care-giver or you yourself will contradict what you have previously said. Once you start contradicting yourself you break the therapeutic alliance.

As patients fall ill, some suffer and others do not. Since we believe that the relief of suffering is one of the primary goals of medicine, it is amazing that not only do patients suffer but many actually seem to suffer more as we treat them. In spite of excellent doctors, excellent nurses, excellent social workers, well-meaning technicians, at times patients suffer more from the treatment than they do from the initial illness. Perhaps we can explain some of that.

First, we need to know what suffering is. Eric Cassel published a fine paper, "The Nature of Suffering and the Goals of Medicine," in 1982. Cassel had considered suffering carefully (also Cassel 1983). In reviewing the literature, he found that most of the time suffering was equated with pain. He and I and many others now feel that they are not the same. Suffering, according to Cassel (1982), is a state of severe distress experienced by persons when events threaten to destroy the integrity of the person. The events may not even be real; they can, however, be perceived to be real.

Suffering can occur on any one of numerous levels. There is the physical level: the pain, the nausea and vomiting, the breathlessness. It can occur on a psychological level: feelings of helplessness and hopelessness, personality changes. Suffering occurs on a social level: the disruption of the social life, loss of job, changes in relationships; people visiting; dissociation from the groups of identity—clubs, co-workers, and the like. Certainly, it can occur on the spiritual level: the existential problem of the end of one's existence. If we know which factors may be contributing to the suffering, we can begin to address them. But the body should not be left just to the doctors and nurses, and the psychologists and psychiatrists should not be the ones to deal with every problem with emotional aspects. We do not necessarily have to call in the clergy when there is a spiritual matter. The social worker need not be the one to address each social problem. No one person can do it all, but each can keep in touch with the different aspects of suffering, address them when they come up, and communicate with the other involved care-givers.

The distinction between pain and suffering is an important point to emphasize. Pain does not mean suffering, nor does suffering come from pain alone. Pain is one cause of suffering, but even severe pain does not cause suffering if the cause of the pain is understood, the end of the pain is in sight, or the pain will result in a good outcome. A good example is the pain of childbirth. For most women, the pain of childbirth may be severe. Nonetheless, most women do not suffer from it.

In order to anticipate and deal with suffering, we have to understand the response of a patient to a chronic illness. Despite our knowing intellectually what it means to have a serious or catastrophic illness, such knowledge is not part of our being. The person who *has* it does not integrate it right away. Patients who have not been chronically ill before, who have had only acute illnesses that respond to medications and disappear, have no experience in dealing with chronic illness. Chronic illness is totally different (Hogshead 1978). We would love to see our patients adjust to chronic illness, to accept the reality of their progressive deterioration. But that does not always happen. More patients accommodate than not; they seem to make some room to tolerate a change in their condition. We can share our thoughts with patients. We can share the patients' thoughts and the patients' feelings—but it is very difficult and it takes a very special alliance between the patient who is ill and the health care worker to get into true feelings of the soul, or the spirit, let alone the thoughts of that patient. When it happens it is wonderful, but it is a very difficult relationship to achieve.

Often, however, patients' perspective on death changes as they get sicker. It changes from the intellectual knowledge, "I have AIDS and I'm probably going to die from this illness," eventually to a point when it becomes more meaningful and real and then becomes integrated. Many patients will tell us that death is actually not the worst alternative. To them the physical suffering and the psychological suffering are really not tolerable anymore.

I think that our attempts to understand some of the emotional realities of dying are doomed to failure if we cling to our old beliefs. Our information about the emotional aspects of what it is like to die is based on primarily anecdotal data. Many of us in the health care field have great difficulty dealing with the fact that someone our own age or younger, someone who is in our peer group, is actually dying. They might be angry with us, we are angry with them. They are not responding to our therapy. It is a very complicated interaction, with transference and countertransference—those words are useful to me even though I am not a psychiatrist—and sometimes we call it inappropriate behavior when the patients are angry with us. We have to allow for that, not take it personally, and realize that we as health care providers can have the same feelings that patients have. Frequently, when we become angry with a patient it is a clue that the patient is also angry. We are sensing that feeling and responding.

I would like to turn to the dying process itself. The dying process is complicated. We can learn from our patients who are dying and use what we learn to help the next patient who faces the threat of death.

Certain fears are seen repeatedly in dying patients. One fear is of the indignity of dying. Patients frequently lose bowel control and are incontinent. They are messy. They have disfiguring lesions. They no longer want to be seen. They are ashamed of how they look or smell. Second, patients fear pain and other symptoms. Too often, patients fear abandonment, and in fact subtle forms of abandonment happen over and over again. We read about it in the newspaper when a child with AIDS is not allowed to go to school. We read studies that describe nurses taking twice as long to answer call lights from patients who are dying of cancer. These are forms of abandonment, and the patients feel it. Patients also fear their nonexistence. I certainly cannot speak much about nonexistence, but it is an area that is useful to address. Patients fear what is going to happen to them after they die.

Mary Baines, a physician who works at St. Christopher's Hospice in London, has further elaborated some of the specific fears, each of which is amenable to therapy. Patients fear not only their symptoms but, more importantly, the significance of their symptoms (Baines

1982). Does bad breath mean I have a recurrence of my lung cancer? Does shortness of breath mean my pneumocystis has returned? Does a new or different pain mean that my disease is progressing? Any new symptom or change in symptom that arises must be addressed in a professional manner and not just brushed aside. Reevaluation and then clear explanation of each new problem and its meaning will do a great deal to allay this set of fears and do a great deal toward helping the patient feel better. Often simple problems are found to be trivial when placed in proper perspective. The shortness of breath, for example, may have been due to bronchitis and the new pain may be only heartburn.

Patients fear that doctors and nurses will not have the skills to help them (Baines 1982). This is often seen when an illness is becoming worse. Patients will ask themselves, "If I had gone to a different doctor, or to a different hospital, would I be in this fix I'm in now?" That is a very difficult situation to deal with: Realize that patients may be thinking along these lines when they start to get angry and start to question you and your treatments.

I have already mentioned the fears of isolation and disfigurement and loss of biological control such as bowel or bladder function. Patients also fear further loss of control. They lose control of their finances. They lose control of their jobs, their environment, and some of the choices in the care they get. We must try our best to give some of it back to those patients. Persons who were functional, active, bright, and responsible citizens are given a diagnosis of AIDS or cancer and suddenly they are "victims" of their disease—such public media and private references to sick people take away their sense of control. Even before there is a drastic change in their health, others are doing things for them that patients are capable of doing themselves. Family and friends try to help out, but instead foster illness behavior.

We can help by giving patients back some power. Let them control their medications when feasible. Include them in decisions about their health, jobs, and finances. Ask intelligent questions and participate in meaningful discussions about their life and illness, but also about ordinary activities of daily life, discussions you would have with a healthy person. Do not patronize people just because they are ill. If we are attuned to these problems, we can help patients merely by treating them as the normal people they are who happen to be ill.

Symptoms of fear can be dealt with humanely when the care-giver has patience and sensitivity to the existence of their symptoms. Depression in someone who is terminally ill, however, is a complex phenomenon. Although superficially it may seem reasonable to accept the depression as appropriate for a person who is dying, I feel this view is incomplete. Many persons spend the last months of life composed, alert, and coping with their illness with an affect that is normal. Others, however, are quite depressed. It is difficult at times to distinguish between the depression that is appropriate for an illness, for which psychosocial intervention is likely to be helpful, and an endogenous or major depression that may require pharmacological intervention in addition to psychotherapy. Needless to say, the vegetative signs of depression are not very helpful diagnostically, as they also may be the symptoms of physical deterioration. How do we distinguish between patients who are depressed and physically ill and those who are just physically ill? Jimmie Holland, who has looked at this question, suggests that if the degree of vegetative signs seems out of proportion to the stage of disease, consider a superimposed depression (Massie, Holland 1984). This takes experience, of course. Keep in mind that as researchers look more closely at adult populations, it is becoming clear that a significant proportion of people suffer from depression. A similar percentage of physically ill persons would be expected to be depressed independent of the illness. I have found it useful to use antidepressant drugs as the nighttime hypnotic when I suspect depression, and get a lot of mileage from a drug such as doxepin with its many desirable properties.

Baines (1982) has looked at depression in the dying patient from a practical and functional perspective. She divides the causes of depression into the categories of past memories, present worries, future fears, and the existential dimension. Past memories include unresolved grief rekindled by the present illness, relationships that have been left unsettled, and guilt from submerged or unfinished issues. Present worries include physical symptoms and their meanings, changes in body image, and the fear of becoming a burden on others. But boredom, financial problems, isolation (overt and implied), and loss of identity as a person are very important as well. Future fears include fear of pain and fears around dying itself, some of which are rational and some not. Fear about an afterlife may be lurking below the surface. Although none of us can fully clarify this issue for the patient, once again anticipating that the issue may lie hidden and opening a door for discussion is often helpful. Lastly, the existential problem of the meaning of one's own life may require examination. Many people fear that their lives have been useless and now no time is left for change. Sometimes guiding patients and families to look at the good that is present in every life helps. Reframing any negative aspects may also prove possible.

There are specific ways that I would like to recommend to help us take better care of patients who are chronically ill and/or dying. These suggestions are from Solomon Papper, a very well-known physician/researcher who died of multiple myeloma. Papper, I feel, left a valuable legacy in a paper in which he discussed with great insight his own illness (1985). I strongly recommend this well-written paper. Papper tells us that, first, we need the knowledge and skills adequate to helping our patients. We have to be confident in our knowledge. We need to keep up with new information. We must know our limits and when to seek help. We have to communicate this explicitly and implicitly to our patients. Fortunately and unfortunately, in San Francisco much information is available, and many of us are almost inundated with continually arriving new data.

Second, we must have clinical creativity. We must have flexibility. We cannot cling to old ideas. What do I mean by that? Diagnostic and therapeutic goals should be set according to the needs of the patient, not according to our old models. Every patient with shortness of breath does not need a new chest X-ray, sputum analysis, and Gallium scan. Incorporate the patient into the decision-making team, so that at least you know that the decisions you make will be what the patient feels is the best decision for him. Give the patient the clinical data. Interpret the data. Explain its significance. And then discuss any tests and what you hope to gain from each one. If doing a new bronchoscopy will allow you the opportunity to treat a person with pneumocystis and treat the shortness of breath, then do it. But if the patient is near death, it is not a procedure I would consider. Again, however, incorporate the patient in the decision-making process.

What you will do, how aggressive you will be, will depend on the clinical stage of the patient's illness. Keep that in mind. A patient who is near death and having diarrhea does not need parasite analysis to document the cause of the diarrhea: Just treat it symptomatically.

Next, Papper tells us to have a meaningful relationship with the patient. No matter how much we care, we can never fully understand what is going on with that patient. But we can try. We can be clear, we can be open, we can listen for clues and cues, and we can at least project the idea that we *want* to hear. Body language should be appropriate and not suggest that we are uncomfortable or in a hurry. We should allow adequate time for our visits so that we can talk with the patient and relate in a meaningful and nonsuperficial way. Many of us have been told in medical school, "Don't get involved with the patient. You will lose your objectivity." Well, needless to say, that is ridiculous. We *are* intimately involved with these patients. There is nothing more intimate than sharing a patient's dying process. It is an honor, a privilege, to be there with that patient, and we have to respect the person who is the patient. They know more about how the experience feels.

Pay attention to details. Papper reminds us how very excited we are to give good news: "The disease is in remission." We call the patient right up and say, "Hey, I've got great news for you." But when the news is not so good, we tend to procrastinate. We tend to be slow to deliver it. If you tell a patient you are going to call Tuesday afternoon with test results, call on Tuesday afternoon. If the test results are not available, call with that information. If you do not, the delay will be interpreted as bad news.

Pay attention to minor symptoms. Address and anticipate other aspects of the care of that patient. Give the patient guidelines for how much time should be spent in bed, how much time up, how much rest is needed, and how much exercise; what the sexual activity level should be; what to eat and not to eat; what is the communicability of the disease. Anticipate these questions. If you see many patients with similar problems, draw up a list to hand out to avoid having to go over every one each time. But still be ready to listen.

Papper also talks about the relationship of the physician, the nurse, social worker, or other provider to the family of the patient. Of course, when I say family, I mean lovers, friends, and significant others as well. Support the friends of the patient. This relationship is not really addressed often, but the same ideas hold. They suffer, too. They often do not know what to say or what not to say. We have the recurring experience in Hospice that the patient says, "I don't want to bother my wife because it will just upset her if she knows I'm dying." And the wife will say, "I don't want to tell my husband that he's going to die. It will upset him." Thus, though they both know the truth, communication, with the opportunity to finish business and express feelings, is blocked.

Our role may be to tell each what the other knows. We can open up communication and see real movement in their relationship even though it is over only a short period of time. Allow all concerned to be care-givers, to be involved. Allow them to do what they can. Teach them to give a bed bath. That is not difficult. Let them touch the patient, get over the fears of touching the patient.

Look at the relationship of the patient to the patient's environment, at the hospital or in the home. What does the room look like? Can we make it more comfortable and livable? How are the ancillary staff, the janitors, the X-ray technicians, relating to the patient? If these relations can all be improved, then they indirectly help the patient.

Lastly—although Papper does not talk about this—I think it is very important to consider the relationship of the care-givers to one another. Who supports the care-givers? Who supports the physicians at San Francisco General who are watching people younger than they are dying of AIDS? Who supports the nurses who are taking care of those patients? We must have support systems, formal and informal, for ourselves as well as for the patients, families, and friends.

Care of the person with AIDS requires that attention be paid to biological, psychological, social, and spiritual aspects of the patient. No matter what the particular area of interest of the care-giver might be, he or she must be familiar with each aspect. Meaningful interventions begin at the time the diagnosis is made and the bad news is delivered. Patients respond differently, according to their underlying personalities, coping strategies, and past experiences with illness and loss. Some may grieve or suffer, others may become depressed or angry, and others may seem unchanged.

To care adequately for the whole person with AIDS, care-givers must have adequate skills and up-to-date information and must be clinically creative and flexible. They must share the decision making with the patient, establish a meaningful relationship with the patient and his significant others, and be able to support other care-givers as well.

References

Baines, M. 1982. The treatment of symptoms in the dying patient. Paper presented at the fourth International Seminar on Terminal Care, October 4–6. Montreal, Quebec.

Cassell, E. J. 1982. The nature of suffering and the goals of medicine. *N Engl J Med* 306:639–45.

———. 1983. The relief of suffering. *Arch Intern Med* 143:522–23.

Garfield, C. 1978. On caring, doctors and death. In *Psychosocial care of the dying patient*, ed. C. Garfield, 3–8. New York: McGraw-Hill Book Co.

Hogshead, H. P. 1978. The art of delivering bad news. In *Psychosocial care of the dying patient*, 128–29, ed. C. Garfield. New York: McGraw-Hill Book Co.

Massie, J. M., and J. C. Holland. 1984. Diagnosis and treatment of depression in the cancer patient. *J Clin Psychiatry* 45:25–28.

Papper, S. 1985. Care of patients with incurable, chronic neoplasm. One patient's perspective. *Am J Med* 78:271–76.

PART II

Mental Health Treatment

7

The Impact of AIDS on the Physician

WILLIAM HORSTMAN AND LEON MCKUSICK

An unexpected change began to occur in our psychotherapy practice several years into the AIDS epidemic. Competent health practitioners who were gay were coming in with similar symptoms: two just out of residency, a physician, dentist, and psychiatrist all with many years of experience working with gay men in private practice.

All these men displayed the set of symptoms that we now describe as the "Helper Helplessness Syndrome." Two were acutely depressed and actively suicidal. One was unable to get out of bed in the morning to go to work. Others were experiencing career dissatisfaction, AIDS-related phobia, nightmares, and anxiety, hopelessness, and general feelings of personal inadequacy. As persistent stressors, the loss of friends and patients to AIDS and their inability as healers to do a thing about it agonized all of them. These men needed a vacation from contact with AIDS patients while they explored their own problems. They had to give up the notion of a practice with patients that were fun to treat; they had to grieve the passing of their own youth and dismiss the self-perception of physician omnipotence.

The projection of the healing doctor was taking a beating, as evidenced by these men. Angry patients and a ridiculing local press in San Francisco were critical of the role of organized medicine. At the same time their training as physicians had effectively discouraged these practitioners from expressing signs of self-doubt in the crisis. As a result, we saw symptoms in these men of what used to be called "combat fatigue" and is now recognized as post-traumatic stress disorder. Unlike the stressors that lead to such diagnosis, however, the trauma causing this distress is unlikely to go away for some time, perhaps not for years. These doctors painfully realized that if they were to continue treating gay men, AIDS would have to be less in their consciousness in order to decrease their depression, anxiety, and ennui. Post-traumatic stress disorder can occur as early as six months after a trauma, but a typical delayed form begins several years following initial exposure to the traumatic events. The latter type describes the condition of our health practitioner patients. The psychological casualties of this disease now included professionals who deal with AIDS as a substantial part of their practice and have difficulty in adjusting to it.

A Study of Physicians

Our observations of this new manifestation of stress disorder led us to investigate the effect on a sample of San Francisco physicians who treat patients with AIDS or ARC in order to understand normative coping strategies for those not in psychotherapy. Of 150 San Francisco Bay Area physicians engaged in AIDS-related professional activity whom we sampled, 82 (55 percent) returned our questionnaire. It was a survey of attitudes toward HIV testing and of psychological reactions to working with AIDS. Forty also consented to be interviewed. Eleven who were not currently working with AIDS patients were excluded from data analysis.

The average age of these seventy-seven male and five female physicians was forty-two. Of them, 33 percent identified themselves as heterosexual, and 63 percent indicated that they were gay or lesbian. One respondent was bisexual, and two physicians refrained from identifying their sexual orientation. Of the entire sample, 31 percent were married, 29 percent lived with partners in primary committed relationships, 13 percent lived apart from primary committed partners, and 26 percent reported not being in a primary relationship. In professional specialties, 29 percent were internists, 26 percent psychiatrists, 12 percent engaged in family or general practice, 6 percent were oncologists, and 5 percent dermatologists. The remaining 22 percent were equally divided among the specialties of gastroenterology, infectious disease, neurology, pathology, clinical microbiology, immunology, public health, anesthesiology, and ophthalmology. The average length of time of working with AIDS was 3.2 years. Mean percent of weekly professional patient contact time with AIDS or ARC was 44.

Psychological Reactions

We assessed in self-report questionnaires the degree of depression, anxiety, overwork, stress, fear of death, intellectual stimulation, and

Table 7.1. *Psychological Reactions of Physicians Working with AIDS*

Since beginning to work with AIDS the physicians (in percentages):

	Have experienced this more or much more than before	Have experienced this about the same amount as before	Have experienced this less or feel it less often
Depression	36	43	21
Anxiety	44	42	14
Overwork	39	42	19
Stress	56	34	11
Fear of death	46	34	20
Intellectual stimulation	46	49	5
Career satisfaction	45	40	15

career satisfaction experienced by these physicians since they had begun working with AIDS.

The majority (56 percent) reported more stress, and a significant minority reported more fear of death (46 percent) and anxiety (44 percent) since they had begun working with AIDS. (See table 7.1.) Paradoxically, more than 40 percent of the sample said that contact with the AIDS epidemic had led to increased intellectual stimulation and career satisfaction.

Differences Between Sample Subgroups

Not surprisingly, we found that physicians who identified themselves as gay are more likely than their heterosexual counterparts to have experienced increased anxiety ($\chi^2=7.4$, df=1, p<.01), overwork ($\chi^2=3.6$, df=1, p<.05), stress ($\chi^2=6.1$, df=1, p<.01), and fear of death ($\chi^2=4.3$, df=1, p<.05) since first working with AIDS. Through interviews, we determined that this differing psychological response is a result of the gay physician's self-perception as being at risk for AIDS, accompanied by identification with an ever increasing number of gay patients whose health status is deteriorating, without having adequate treatment alternatives.

In general, the high-risk sexual behavior of gay men has decreased dramatically since the epidemic became noticeable (McKusick, Horstman, Coates 1985, McKusick, Wiley, Coates 1985). The behavior of gay physicians is no exception. More are single and hence more at risk than their heterosexual colleagues. Both gay and heterosexual doctors have experienced differences in relationship status and change in number of sexual partners since their work with AIDS began. (See table 7.2.) Of particular interest is the high percentage of safe sex practices for the heterosexual physicians. One thirty-two-year-old family practitioner interpreted this data quite poignantly when she said, "Seeing so many men die simply from having sex has given me second thoughts about any man putting any of his fluid in me for any reason unless I decide to have kids, and then I'm going to be damn sure we are both antibody-negative." Even with no rational reason to believe that they had been exposed to AIDS, other heterosexual physicians described diminished interest in sex. They made irrational associations between all forms of sexual expression and AIDS before the psychological relief they felt upon receiving negative HIV antibody test results.

Sexual partners and practices and emotional relationships were just some of the worries we encountered. Some gay physicians, for example, were concerned about becoming publicly known as homosexual because of their interest in AIDS and therefore being discriminated against. One resident described this episode:

> I was working in the intensive care unit with my team, none of whom knew I was gay. A young man was brought in who had a diagnosis of PC [*Pneumocystis carinii*] pneumonia and CNS lymphoma. He looked up at me and said: "Didn't we fuck last Christmas?" I took a second look at him and asked myself, "Where was I last Christmas?" After I picked my mouth up off the floor, I said to my team, "We need to determine his change in mental status."

Other studies have found generally the highest stress in those physicians conducting solo practice (Mawardi 1983). In our study, openly gay physicians in well-established private practices worried less about public exposure of their sexual identity but were much more likely to experience grief because they had developed personal relationships with their patients:

> Most of the patients I have known for years. I used to have two deaths a year. Now I have two a month. I just lost one yesterday. I had saved him

Table 7.2. *Differences Between Gay and Heterosexual Physicians on Life-style and Sexual Behavior Variables*

	Gay (%)	Heterosexual (%)
Relationship status		
Married	2	80
Committed relationship, living together	43	5
Committed relationship, living apart	20	5
Single	35	10
Change in numbers of sexual partners		
Remains monogamous or celibate	12	70
Has become monogamous or celibate	32	10
Has reduced numbers of partners	48	5
Has maintained the same number of partners	8	15
Amount of safe sex (no-body-fluid-exchange)		
No sex at all	4	0
Only safe sex	42	47
Mostly safe sex	46	7
Some safe sex	4	7
No safe sex	4	40

from PCP a year ago. He had full confidence I was going to save him again. I didn't live up to his expectations. His brother said, "You gave him a year." It put me to tears.

Physicians in private practice trained in family or general practice or internal medicine have been forced to become adept at treating very sick people with a myriad of life-threatening illnesses. One forty-seven-year-old internist who had been in private practice for fourteen years told us, "The stress is just like medical school, only worse, and I can't imagine another twenty years of this."

The five women physicians we interviewed were much less personally threatened by AIDS since none was a risk group member. Before the beginning of the epidemic, three of these five women had had a number of gay male patients who specifically sought them out because they were more comfortable seeing a woman physician for medical or psychiatric problems. As a group, these physicians reported more professional isolation, less dissatisfaction with their practices, and less stress. One lesbian resident quipped, "For a lesbian, any sex is safe sex." Therefore, she of all respondents is least likely to experience contagion anxiety. Because she identifies with gay men, she feels a missionary zeal about AIDS and plans to make AIDS medicine her special focus.

All medical specialties and levels of training are affected by the AIDS crisis. Medical residents in San Francisco are subjected to their own set of problems with respect to AIDS. Because of the already high levels of stress that residents experience, respondents reported higher levels of distaste for AIDS patients as well as describing homophobic sentiment in other residents, particularly Caucasian heterosexual men. A number of explanations were offered for this dynamic.

The "desirable" disease was described by one resident as one that is curable, has a "high-tech" diagnosis or treatment, and is nonchronic. The preferred patient is one who is intelligent enough to comply with directives but not too questioning and challenging, and from the same cultural background as the resident. From a disease standpoint, AIDS is seen as undesirable, since persons with AIDS require an immense amount of care and attention with poor prognoses and no high-tech cure available. As patients, persons with AIDS are attractive to all but heterosexual male residents, possibly because of the age similarity and the threat of identification with a homosexual who is typically intelligent enough to ask probing questions. One specific territorial dispute had erupted at San Francisco General Hospital when the expansion of the AIDS inpatient unit threatened to displace residents to more cramped sleeping quarters. As one respondent remarked, "You should never come between a resident and his four hours of nightly sleep."

Ways of Coping with Stress

When asked according to a pretested checklist how they cope with the emotional aspects of working with AIDS, our respondents cited talking to friends, lovers, or family members as the most likely ways to reduce the stress, and negative stress reduction techniques such as

Table 7.3. Ways Physicians Cope with AIDS-Related Stress (%)

66	Talk to a friend, lover, or family member
65	Teach others about AIDS
54	Remain objective
48	Get support from other physicians
42	Exercise
37	Spend time quietly
34	Get depressed
27	Involved in hobbies
25	Get angry
25	Limit the number of hours in AIDS work
21	Cry
16	Engage in spiritual activities
14	Don't think about it
14	Go to a psychotherapist
13	Drink alcohol
11	Have sex
1	Take a pill

taking a pill, having sex, or drinking alcohol as the least likely ways. (See table 7.3.)

Although about half of the sample relied on other physicians for support, few in the interviews expressed any motivation or desire to attend support groups composed of physicians to discuss AIDS-related stress. As one doctor put it, "Why get together with a bunch of other doctors and have a bitch session? My life is bad enough." Many believed that talking about AIDS after work made the emotional impact worse.

In the interviews, many physicians reported reduced drug and alcohol use since both drugs and alcohol increase psychological distress and decrease immune functioning. As a group, these physicians have made specific behavioral changes such as altering sexual practices, reducing drug and alcohol use, and developing coping strategies in order to stay healthy and minimize psychological impact. Effectively handling stressful situations, however, is contingent on both what one

Table 7.4. Changes in Drug and Alcohol Use Since First Working with AIDS

	The respondent has (by %):			
	Never used this or stopped	Reduced	Maintained same level	Increased
Alcohol	17	15	65	3
Minor tranquilizers	69	9	20	3
Drugs for recreation	63	26	11	0

Table 7.5. Physicians' Future Projections About the Epidemic

Percent of physicians who believe:

	Within 1 year	1–5 years	5–10 years	More than 10 years	Don't know
An AIDS vaccine will be ready for the general population	0	31	41	11	17
The number of new cases of AIDS per month will not increase in San Francisco	9	55	22	10	4

Percent of physicians who believe:

	Less than 4000	4000 to 7000	7000 to 10,000	10,000 to 15,000	More than 15,000	Don't know
The number of cumulative cases of AIDS to expect in San Francisco by 1990	4	30	24	18	10	14

does behaviorally in response to the stress (tables 7.2, 7.3, and 7.4) and one's ability to handle the variability—in this case, of the clinical picture of AIDS itself. Will the epidemic decrease or increase? When will it end? Physicians are particularly vulnerable to these questions because their training, their patients, and the public demand concrete answers.

Our data showed a relationship between reported level of subjective distress and tolerance for uncertainty in estimating the duration and severity of the epidemic. (See table 7.5.) Whereas we did not find a relationship between increased stress and negative future projections about numbers of cases or epidemic severity, we did find that those who were less likely to report stress were also more likely to respond "I don't know" when asked about expected numbers of future AIDS cases. Increased stress in an ambiguous situation can cause the physician, by virtue of his intellect and training, to make assertions based on existing evidence that may very well be untrue. Those who are more capable of tolerating the ambiguity of the unknown by simply saying "I don't know" may be subjecting themselves, and perhaps others, to less stress by their conservatism.

Correlates of AIDS Burnout

The higher percentage of time a physician spends in contact with AIDS patients, the more likely he or she is to experience psychological distress, as defined by our measures. The number of years spent working with AIDS does not correlate with psychological distress, although percentage of inpatient time per week with AIDS patients is related to depression ($\chi^2=4.3$, df=1, p<.05), overwork ($\chi^2=6.6$, df=1, p<.01), as well as intellectual stimulation ($\chi^2=5.5$, df=1, p<.05). AIDS practitioner burnout appears to be a function less of longitudinal contact with the disease than of concentrated exposure. This was exemplified by one of our gay respondents, who stated: "As a doctor, I have an inner conviction that excites me and drives me at times at my own expense."

It seems reasonable that inpatient time working with AIDS would correlate with depression and overwork. Few of our inpatient physicians had much prior exposure to the terminally ill in such numbers. Almost all expressed the value of oncological training or the wish that it had been their subspecialty, since "oncologists deal with deadly disease all the time and go in with their eyes wide open."

AIDS burnout has its own set of patient/doctor dynamics that needs to be assessed by any mental health professional working in close collaboration with the AIDS physician. Frequently, he or she may be angry in countertransference to the patient because he or she is incapable of doing anything beyond giving symptomatic relief. One physician explained his relief when a patient dies: "I don't have to deal anymore with the complaints that I couldn't do anything about anyway. It's also easier to accept his death if I'm mad at him because there is safety in that kind of distance from a patient."

Similarly, certain types of patients have been found especially distasteful to some of our respondents. Hypochondriacal men who want reassurance and do not respond to commonsense advice are particularly taxing to AIDS primary care physicians: "It's the neurotic psychosomatic patient I can't stand. After a day of trying to save dying men, when someone comes in obsessed with a pimple, I find myself wanting to shout 'Will you grow up? Don't you know people are dying?'"

Aside from the negative psychological impact AIDS has had on these physicians, it has increased intellectual and career satisfaction as well as elevating some to professional success, as experienced by a thirty-six-year-old married heterosexual man: "The AIDS epidemic has given me the opportunity for success, to distinguish me from the next Joe. I had a very successful father and brother. This has allowed me the expression of my persona that has satisfied me."

Another thirty-six-year-old heterosexual man describes how AIDS attracts the young doctor with a social conscience:

> Young physicians who have recently finished their training are attracted to this disease. There is space in their schedule to tackle it: After you have been in academic medicine for five years either you have failed or your time is committed. It attracts a socially conscious group of doctors. I was politicized in the antiwar movement of the sixties and then by being a man close to the women's movement, so I was more prepared to react to this disease without prejudice.

Although we have described the psychological hazards of working with AIDS, we need also to acknowledge the intellectual stimulation AIDS provides, the potentiality for a deepened understanding of profound aspects of the human condition. Many of these doctors are highly dedicated and principled people who were aware of the importance of their work and were deriving satisfaction from performing it to the best of their training and personal abilities.

Implications for Mental Health Professionals

Mental health professionals can learn from these physicians about the importance of becoming aware of the causes of burnout and then acting to limit their own battle fatigue in their work with AIDS.

A simple remedy for AIDS-related burnout is reflected by this physician's report: "I get away on vacation more often, far enough away to realize how depressed everyone is in San Francisco and how the rest of the world is still going along as usual." Periodic getaways break the insulating effect of working in an epidemic, divert the practitioner to other mental stimulation, and freshen emotional resources.

The majority of these professionals find it easier to cope by confiding in friends or spouses, by teaching others about AIDS and, most interestingly, by remaining objective. Many of us in mental health would rather avoid placing an objective guise on intellectual distance, which can isolate us from our clients. Refraining from overidentification, however, can protect us from feeding on the crises of those we help. Presenting the most objective, nonbiased, up-to-date factual information during therapy has helped to limit anxiety and hysteria. This places a responsibility on mental health professionals to become, and remain, well informed about medical developments associated with AIDS.

Second, we can use our skills to help physicians as they cope with this disease, trading our expertise in human psychology for their medical knowledge. As we seek a therapeutic alliance with someone who has AIDS or ARC, we quickly become aware of allied medical professionals with whom our client has contact, and we become aware of his host of anxieties, attitudes, and emotions toward medicine and toward the primary or AIDS physician. Understanding and interpreting anger and dissatisfaction at the quality of medical help available will be one of our tasks. Mediation by the therapist between patient and doctor has also smoothed the course of treatment for many persons with AIDS, discouraging acting out of angry feelings by both parties. We can make it our responsibility to keep the doctors at the bedsides of our clients with AIDS.

As we work with a person coping with AIDS, we soon become aware of the whole institution of medicine fighting to cope with AIDS: the neurologist at a case conference confessing that the disease has overwhelmed the resources of his department; the private physician treating our patient, angry and frustrated at having to fill out lengthy reports required by the government for each new AIDS patient, without reimbursement, only to help the body count go higher;

the researcher who is besieged with requests by persons with AIDS who want to be part of the drug trial he is designing, caught between his objective criteria and his desire to help. At first, most of us may need to adjust our image of the benevolent and powerful medical profession well prepared for all crises, realizing that stress has penetrated medical practice and that those doctors also at work on our cases may need occasional impromptu psychological consultation. Insofar as we are trained to ease human suffering and psychological difficulty, we may find our skills very handy in helping those physicians with whom we come in contact—in small but essential ways—to cope.

References

Mawardi, B. W. 1983. Aspects of the impaired physician. In *Stress and burnout in the human services profession*, ed. B. A. Farber, 119–27. New York: Pergamon Press.

McKusick, L., W. R. Horstman, and T. J. Coates. 1985. AIDS and the sexual behavior reported by gay men in San Francisco. *Am J Public Hlth* 75: 493–96.

McKusick, L., J. Wiley, T. J. Coates, et al. 1985. Reported changes in the sexual behavior of men at risk for AIDS, San Francisco, 1982–84: The AIDS Behavioral Research Project. *Pub Hlth Rep* 100 (6): 622–29.

8

Psychosocial Challenges of AIDS and ARC: Clinical and Research Observations

JEFFREY S. MANDEL

One of the most striking and recurring themes that clinicians encounter in working with persons with AIDS and ARC is the struggle to maintain hope. Helping people with life-threatening illnesses always presents a difficult challenge, but for many clinicians assisting those with AIDS or ARC is a particularly complex task. Often our patients' hopes and concerns arise from several overlapping areas. To understand these fully, we must consider not only the traditional approaches to treating those with life-threatening illness but also the unhappy fact that so much remains unknown about AIDS.

In addition, AIDS has become a powerful sociocultural event that involves mass hysteria, political and scientific battles resulting in conflicting information, and a long history of association between homosexuality and mental illness. Another powerful and complicating element is the problem of countertransference—clinicians may see their own fears of life-threatening illness reflected and then played out. All these elements of the AIDS environment complicate attempts to keep hope alive.

This overview of psychosocial challenges affecting persons with ARC and those recently diagnosed with AIDS and the treatment issues that arise from them is drawn from clinical and research sources: the experiences of several clinical practitioners in the San Francisco Bay Area and the preliminary findings of ongoing psychosocial research by members of the Biopsychosocial AIDS Project at the University of California, San Francisco (UCSF-BAP).

According to the model we adopted for researching and treating AIDS (Coates, Temoshok, Mandel 1984), biological, psychological, and social spheres of influence are understood as being in constant interaction. Thus it is impossible to have a significant impact on one sphere without also affecting the others. As AIDS affects our culture, so our culture affects an individual's experience of AIDS.

A Longitudinal Psychosocial Study of Persons with AIDS and ARC

In UCSF-BAP's primary five-year psychosocial study of persons with AIDS and ARC, sponsored by the National Institute of Mental Health (NIMH), researchers working with Lydia Temoshok, principal investigator of this study, document the psychosocial impact and consequences of events that occur along the continuum of AIDS viral infections and treatment. The perspective of the study is longitudinal. The gay men with AIDS and ARC who volunteered to participate in the study are interviewed two to eight weeks after diagnosis, and at four, seven, and fifteen months after the initial interview. At each point, researchers assess medical status and administer a structured interview and self-report package. Because the interviews have been conducted exclusively with gay men, this presentation is directed chiefly to clinicians who work with this group. Nevertheless, most of the findings are applicable to other populations as well.

Reactions to Diagnosis

The study has documented how individuals react to their diagnoses of AIDS or ARC (Mandel 1985). Affective reactions to AIDS or ARC among the study participants soon after diagnosis were further contrasted with reactions of a matched group of men diagnosed with malignant melanoma—this latter group of men was interviewed and given similar self-report instruments in an earlier study (Temoshok 1985). Among three groups, we found a highly similar range of reactions in the two-month period following diagnosis. All groups showed mean clinical levels of distress, anxiety, and depression. (See next chapter.)

In a similar study conducted by William Woods (1985), a member of the UCSF-BAP research team, results from the NIMH study were corroborated. Woods contrasted the psychological status of four groups of men—with AIDS-associated KS soon after diagnosis; with acute leukemia soon after diagnosis; and two control groups: one of apparently healthy gay-identified men and the other of healthy heterosexual men. Those with KS and acute leukemia, as well as the healthy gay-identified men, were similar to one another on measures of depression, anxiety, distress, and locus of control. They were more dysphoric, however, than the group of healthy heterosexual men. As in our NIMH longitudinal study, mean dysphoria scores for the KS, acute leukemia, and healthy gay groups were at clinical levels. What these studies suggest is that these men experience a typical human response to life-threatening illness.

The unexpected finding that healthy gay-identified men shared high levels of emotional distress with their sick gay and heterosexual counterparts reveals the powerful impact of the AIDS epidemic on those at high risk for the disease. Healthy individuals who experience profound psychosocial dilemmas as a result of the AIDS epidemic may need interventions to help them cope with their distress. This may be even more crucial if psychosocial variables are found to be implicated as cofactors in disease onset or progression.

Assessment of Mood or Cognitive Disturbance

With AIDS or ARC, complications emerge in assessing mood or cognitive disturbances because emotional states follow the medical course of the diseases—unpredictable and fluctuating. Fatigue, a common symptom of AIDS, for example, can also be a symptom of chronic anxiety or depression. Among physically sick patients, the experience of distress or dysphoria is likely to have both biological and psychosocial determinants.

Conversely, psychosocial factors may affect the perception of physical symptoms. As clinicians, we encounter a common problem in distinguishing between physical symptoms of AIDS and hypochondriasis. Patients with ARC report having particular difficulty in getting their health care providers to take their concerns seriously. Founded upon denial of emotional conflict, hypochondriasis may permit patients to express their concerns more comfortably—not only about physical symptoms but also about the adequacy of health care.

Another confounding factor is the possibility of organic problems. (See chapters by Wolcott and Tucker above.) Overall, researchers and clinicians have begun to pay increasing attention to the neurotropic nature of HIV. Organic involvement can have profound effects upon mood *and* cognition; thus it can frighten and confuse patient and clinician alike.

Although half the men in the NIMH study had sought some form of mental health assistance, unmet needs are great as a result of inadequate resources or of staff or patient beliefs that apparent problems are gay or personal issues that must be dealt with outside traditional settings. In many settings, concerned providers struggle to provide basic medical services; they may not give psychosocial services a high priority.

Our experience in San Francisco suggests, however, that most persons with AIDS or ARC adjust to their diagnosis without disabling psychosocial problems. In fact, most patients develop a very positive spirit. As clinicians, we may be surprised by this positive spirit and hopefulness and interpret it as denial. As a result, we may mistakenly encourage our patients to experience what is assumed to be their real underlying pain—a common error of clinicians with limited experience in working with life-threatening illness. For most persons with AIDS or ARC, quality of life becomes a primary goal, and they quickly become expert at making the most of their precious time.

Attribution: The Search for Meaning

The study also has focused on the theories developed by men with AIDS or ARC about (1) why they developed their health problems and (2) which factors may play a role in the possible improvement of their health. These theories, known as attributions, are important in adjusting to illness because they create understanding and a sense of meaning, mastery, and control. Naturally, individuals form theories about the origins and meaning of their illness. These theories are then related to the kinds of life-style changes they make after being diagnosed.

In this portion of the larger NIMH study, Jeffrey Moulton (n.d.) examined the possible associations between attributions and emotional distress. Among men with AIDS, the attribution of illness to external sources, such as bad luck or the environment, seemed to be emotionally protective. Attributing responsibility to oneself for a life-threatening condition can be devastating. If experienced as a "death warrant," a diagnosis of AIDS may involve blaming one's character or behavior for a condition for which no redress may be available.

Among persons with ARC, a syndrome less likely to be perceived as irreversible or lethal, Moulton did not find the same association between distress and self-attribution. Self-attribution of possible improvements in health (or an individual's belief that he could influence his health status through particular kinds of changes in life-style) was associated with less distress. Feeling that one can or cannot influence the course of illness may be an important factor differentiating those persons with ARC who adapt to the challenge of their health condition from those who become psychosocially disabled.

Moulton (1985) found that postdiagnostic life-style changes—improving diet and exercise, starting various stress-reduction techniques—in addition to their possible healthful effects, may be part of the coping process to restore psychological and social equilibrium. Those men who had made many changes were less distressed or felt more hopeful, on the average, than those who had made few changes. These results indicate that we may find it useful to explore the meaning that our patients seek to find from their illness and to encourage positive changes in them. Some clinicians are in conflict about being openly directive, perhaps especially those of us who have been trained analytically. But dealing with terminal illness requires a shift toward a more active technique.

Social Support and Coping

At all points in the coping process, participants in the study revealed social support to be the most helpful element (Moulton 1985; next chapter). Jane Zich (n.d.), another member of the research team, is finding that among participants soon after diagnosis, emotionally sustaining kinds of social support were more desirable, useful, available, and likely to be used than problem-solving types of support.

An outpouring of social support from services available to these men may have a particularly profound impact on those who had never before experienced such deeply felt acceptance. Social support may answer a long-held yearning by some gay men for acceptance by family, friends, and society. Although tragic in its timing, an AIDS diagnosis may provide some people with their first opportunity to incorporate the experience of caring and return it in kind. The absence of caring services in other localities may be as much a tragedy as their presence is a blessing in the Bay Area.

With the threat of death, psychological processes may become heightened and accelerated. For some men with AIDS or ARC, this increased sensitivity may offer the possibility of an awareness and wisdom beyond their years. I have often been awed by the clarity and power of some of my clients when faced with the challenge of AIDS. The world does not stop with AIDS; indeed much remains possible in the lives of those with AIDS or ARC, and it waits to take shape.

In addition to social support, study participants reported that their own inner resources and spiritual beliefs were of critical importance in dealing with the issues that confronted them after their diagnosis (Moulton 1985). Many men transformed their health problems into a more positive perspective on life. For some, the effect was to increase the value of the "little" things that make life meaningful and pleasurable, such as taking more time to enjoy activities and friends, as well as reassessing values and priorities.

Particularly for persons with AIDS, being diagnosed with a life-threatening illness may prompt profound changes in personality and attitude. Tom Irish, M.A., a member of the team, reports that some of the men described their lives before their AIDS diagnosis as self-serving, competitive, and utilitarian. Afterward, these men began to place primary value on compassion, caring, and spiritual concerns. One study participant remarked, "With the fast-paced life I led before, I don't know if there was any other way for me to learn these things except through AIDS."

Self-Disclosure About Health Problems

Another focus of the study has been on relationships among emotional distress, open discussion of one's health problems, and "coming out" as being gay. Approximately 80 percent of the men in the study had disclosed their homosexuality to their families and to colleagues at work before being diagnosed. Two months after their diagnoses, however, one-third of the men with AIDS and half of the men with ARC had not discussed their health problems with one or more family members or in the workplace. Not having "come out" as a gay man was the most common reason for *not* discussing health problems with others. Most men who did discuss their health problems with others reported a positive experience, while those who chose not to do so reported more distress (Mandel 1985).

Telling others about AIDS-related health problems or concerns forms a necessary bridge between the stress of diagnosis and the development of social support. For both patients and health care providers, dealing with AIDS implies a confrontation with cultural taboos against homosexuality and promiscuity. It is often assumed that the person with AIDS or ARC has a sexually promiscuous life-style (Altman 1986). Such stigmatization can contribute to the patient's sense of isolation, shame, self-blame, or distress (Dilley 1985); or it can reactivate dormant conflicts about sexuality (Solomon, Mead n.d.).

One thorny issue that arises is whether or not to tell one's sexual partners about health problems—or to have sexual relations at all. Some clinicians encourage safe sex as a bottom line; others insist that it is an ethical obligation to tell all partners about health problems. Clients and clinicians bring strong feelings to this issue. All clinicians have an obligation to explore their own feelings about sex and AIDS so as not to burden patients with their own moral or sexual prohibitions. Those who do not find the recommended precautions against contagion adequate or who feel that they cannot endorse accepted safe sex guidelines should request not to be involved with AIDS or ARC patients.

Psychoneuroimmunologic Considerations

The emotional reactions and coping responses of men with AIDS or ARC are obviously important for the quality of their lives. They may also be significant for another very important reason: Emotional experiences may affect the actual immunologic processes that determine health outcomes. Recent research in the field of psychoneuroimmunology has demonstrated the effects of psychological and emotional factors on various aspects of immune function (Ader 1981; Coe, Levine 1986).

An investigation being conducted by members of the NIMH team—Lydia Temoshok, Jane Zich, Daniel Stites, George Solomon, and Anne O'Leary—and supported by the Joan B. Kroc Foundation is an intensive psychoimmunologic study of differences between long-surviving persons with AIDS and a comparison sample of persons with AIDS who are "average" in their medical status. Investigators hope that this study will yield clues about the kinds of psychosocial factors (emotional and behavioral) that may contribute to unusually long survival with AIDS.

Psychoneuroimmunology is commanding the attention of the professional and lay public; it entices us with the hope of personal powerfulness in the absence of effective biomedical treatments for AIDS. There exists no evidence at this time, however, that such factors as stress and depression or expressiveness of emotions are contributing cofactors in AIDS disease progression. Although quality of life is clearly affected by psychosocial variables, length of survival time after diagnosis may prove to be unaffected by such factors.

Studies such as this are important because they emphasize that AIDS need not be a death sentence. Not only are some men alive three or four years after diagnosis but they are living meaningful and productive lives. They appear to be healthy and they report a high degree of well-being. Perceptions of a disease that is necessarily followed by physical decline and death may form a self-fulfilling prophecy; it is difficult to fight such a powerful cultural projection.

Problems in the Definition of ARC

Gradually, public attention has increasingly focused on people who are at risk of AIDS and who *have* conditions apparently related to the immune disorder, but whose conditions are not yet included within the CDC definition of AIDS itself. (See chapter by Abrams above.) For researchers, the lack of a clear and stable definition of ARC* makes it difficult to choose comparable cohorts, confounds interpretation of results, and makes it difficult to compare results among studies. Although ARC surveillance data is just now being collected, available data suggest that only 6 to 25 percent of diagnosed cases of ARC will progress to AIDS (Fishbein et al. 1985). Thus, ARC conditions may reflect a moderate amount of immunocompromise, but not progressive disease. Unfortunately, health officials estimate that ten times as many persons have ARC as have AIDS. But inaccurate case reporting and concerns about confidentiality among physicians and patients compromise ARC (and AIDS) surveillance data.

The men with ARC who volunteered to participate in our NIMH study were identified by their physicians as having two or more signs or symptoms thought to be AIDS-related but falling outside the CDC definition of AIDS. This working definition is quite similar to that proposed by the Bay Area Physicians for Human Rights (BAPHR 1986).

Unrecognized Psychosocial Problems of Persons with ARC

Overall, an emerging theme in the study emphasizes that the psychosocial needs of persons with ARC have been unrecognized and underestimated. Whereas most clinicians are well educated about the signs of AIDS, the earlier signs of ARC are less well known and more diffuse. Because most persons with AIDS first experience ARC symptoms, the following health history factors apply to most in both groups.

---

*As this manuscript was being prepared, the CDC continued its efforts to describe and classify the full spectrum of AIDS viral infection, from seropositivity and asymptomatic infection to initial clinical symptoms to serious opportunistic infections and cancer.

Study participants were asked to describe the first symptom they noticed that they attributed to later development of AIDS or ARC. More than half of the men with ARC had not been concerned about this first symptom or attributed it to something else. Consequently, they did not immediately see a doctor. Many men delayed more than eight months before making a medical appointment. Study participants report that in the first examination their physicians were most likely to tell them that their symptoms were nothing to worry about or that they did not know what the symptoms were.

This initial visit to the doctor may mark the first of many frustrating situations for persons with ARC. To avoid the great uncertainty of the situation, patient and health care provider often collude in denial. With ARC, physicians have few tools except to reassure patients that their conditions are not serious or to try and soothe them by telling them not to worry. For the patients, the reassurance can feel like an invalidation of their fears. Because the uncertainty evokes similar fears in others, friends will often contribute to this "everything will be fine" scenario, rather than empathize with the distress of the person who has the symptoms.

The uncertainty faced by persons with ARC makes it clear why those in the study were even more distressed than those with AIDS. Although most will remain medically stable over time, both the range and intensity of their affective reactions to diagnosis suggest that they are reacting *as if* they had been diagnosed with a life-threatening illness. Persons with ARC who were interviewed more recently, however, were less depressed and less confused than those interviewed up to a year earlier (Temoshok et al. n.d.). Changes in medical response, in the direction of greater specificity and legitimization of ARC as a medical syndrome, may have had a positive psychosocial impact on this group.

Whereas with AIDS, fear of contagion—in the home, workplace, or treatment setting—may be tempered by the sympathy extended to one who has a terminal illness, there may be no such moderating effects for persons with ARC because of the uncertainty about what the diagnosis means. For half of the men with ARC in the study, their illness was severe enough to cause disability or unemployment. Lacking a clear diagnosis, many men feel guilty about taking needed time away from work to recuperate from intermittent illness or to put personal affairs in order. Decisions about leaving work are further complicated by the fact that persons with ARC do not qualify for Social Security benefits; the federal government does not recognize ARC as a disabling condition.

Searching for hope in the absence of definitive medical treatment, persons with ARC, as well as those with AIDS, frequently seek other than mainstream medical treatments. Many physicians discourage or at best tolerate questions about these treatments, inadvertently pushing their patients to rely exclusively on the medical establishment, continue the search for these treatments clandestinely, or reject the medical establishment altogether. Whether or not alternative treatments are of medical value, clinicians should support their patients' searches for hope.

Some physicians, sensing the emotional distress of their patients, suggest that they see mental health professionals. We need to acknowledge that healing can take place not only at a physical level but also at emotional, mental, and spiritual levels (Solomon, Mead 1986). There are many ways of bolstering hope, alternative treatments being but one. At the very least, we should encourage our patients to educate themselves about what is known and to take an active role in their own health care.

Health care providers should be alert particularly to the psychosocial needs of persons with ARC. In order to help people recognize early signs of illness and to encourage changes in behavior that may affect health outcomes, we should specifically target these men through education and prevention programs.

Conclusion

Sometimes people speak of "false hope," but perhaps such a thing really does not exist. Hopelessness is a dangerous place, a place in which people are depressed and withdrawn. As anyone who has worked with terminally ill patients will tell you, it often draws death about itself quickly. Hope, however, is the foundation on which people enhance their health as best they can, draw friends around them, and perhaps even live longer. With the media so full of misleading statements about 100 percent mortality with AIDS, it is crucial that we support those with AIDS or ARC in their struggles to maintain hope. We must recognize that, as clinicians, we are not colluding in our patients' defenses; rather we are supporting something vital to the quality, and maybe even to the length, of their lives.

References

Ader, R., ed. 1981. *Psychoneuroimmunology*. New York: Academic Press.

Altman, D. 1986. *AIDS in the mind of America*. New York: Anchor Press/ Doubleday.

Bay Area Physicians for Human Rights. 1986. Proposed guidelines to define ARC. San Francisco. Typescript.

Coates, T. J., L. Temoshok, and J. S. Mandel. 1984. Psychosocial research is essential to understanding and treating AIDS. *Am Psychologist* 39:1309–14.

Coe, C. L., and S. Levine. 1986. Psychoimmunology: An old idea whose time has come. In *Biological and behavioral correlates of psychopathology*, ed. T. Perez, J. Chiodo, and J. H. Harvey. Vol. 3. Lubbock: Texas Technological University.

Dilley, J., H. Ochitill, M. Perl, et al. 1985. Findings in psychiatric consultations with patients with acquired immune deficiency syndrome. *Am Psychiatrist* 142:82–86.

Fishbein, D. B., J. E. Kaplan, T. J. Spera, et al. 1985. Unexplained lymphadenopathy in homosexual men: A longitudinal study. *JAMA* 254:930–35.

Mandel, J. S. 1985. Affective reactions to a diagnosis of AIDS or ARC in gay men. Ph.D. diss., Wright Institute, Los Angeles.

Moulton, J. M. 1985. Adjustment to a diagnosis of acquired immune deficiency syndrome and related conditions: A cognitive and behavioral perspective. Ph.D. diss., California School of Professional Psychology, Berkeley.

Moulton, J. M., and D. Sweet. n.d. Attributions of cause and improvement among gay men with AIDS and ARC. University of California, San Francisco, Biopsychosocial AIDS Project. Typescript.

Solomon, G. F., and C. W. Mead. n.d. Psychological and psychiatric considerations in the treatment of gay patients with AIDS or ARC. University of California, San Francisco, Biopsychosocial AIDS Project. Typescript.

Temoshok, L., and Biopsychosocial AIDS Project. n.d. Differential psychosocial sequelae in AIDS and ARC. University of California, San Francisco. Typescript.

Temoshok, L., B. W. Heller, R. W. Sagebiel, M. S. Blois, et al. 1985. The relationship of psychosocial factors to prognostic indicators in cutaneous malignant melanoma. *J Psychosocial Res* 29 (2):139–53.

Woods, W. J. 1985. A comparison study of psychological status of AIDS-associated Kaposi's sarcoma patients, acute leukemia patients, and healthy gay and heterosexual men. Ph.D. diss., Ohio State University, Columbus.

Zich, J., and L. Temoshok. n.d. Perceptions of social support in men with AIDS and ARC: Relationships with distress, hardiness, and mortality. University of California, San Francisco, Biopsychosocial AIDS Project. Typescript.

9

Treatment Issues Concerning Persons with AIDS

SHEILA NAMIR

Consider the impact of AIDS on a person's life: He must change life-style and behavior, reexamine his priorities and aspirations, cope with a complex medical system, and establish adequate relationships with care-givers. He often must deal with pain and incapacity and adjust to changes in external reality—relationships with family and friends and lovers, changes in income as well as in livelihood and social roles. He has to work again on issues that were once thought resolved, such as attitudes toward one's own sexuality, dependency needs, reactions to authority figures, and feelings of helplessness.

For many, the traditional means of coping are not available. Their support networks often disappear, and their fears of transmitting the disease to others cause increased isolation. Little conclusive information is available, and talking about the disease often creates more alienation and discrimination. The routine of their lives is seriously disrupted.

It is no wonder that in a recent survey of the needs of persons with AIDS, 81 percent of those surveyed wanted individual or group psychotherapy (Wolcott, Fawzy et al. in press). This was the third greatest service need, following medical information about treatments and information about the causes of AIDS. The survey also indicated that we are not meeting that need, with only 28 percent of respondents receiving even minimal psychological services.

Purposes of Psychological Intervention

The first basic purpose of intervening with someone who has AIDS is to help him come to terms with the diagnosis and its meaning for him. Asking a person "What do you understand about your illness?" elicits a great deal of information, giving the mental health practitioner an opportunity to understand that person's fantasies, attitudes, and concerns about AIDS. Shock, acute anxiety, despair, anger, and sudden withdrawal and isolation are common reactions to a diagnosis of AIDS. A diagnosis also means immediate changes in one's life-style. Often a period of denial is unavailable to a person with AIDS because of the media focus on the disease and because he has known other people with AIDS and assumes that his course will be similar to theirs.

A second goal of intervention is to increase the quality of life. Too often when we intervene in life-threatening illness there is a tendency to concentrate on issues of death and dying and to forget about life and living. A primary focus needs to be "Now that you've been diagnosed with AIDS, how are you going to live your life?" An exploration of changes in one's life, aspirations, priorities, and goals—given a diagnosis of AIDS—provides a framework for adaptation to the illness and for developing new coping strategies or enhancing those that worked previously.

A third goal is to help the person feel more in control rather than feel a helpless, hopeless victim of a disease. Helping to regain or increase the management of his life is crucial here. A medically ill patient can alleviate some feelings of helplessness by understanding cognitively the cause of the illness and learning how to secure appropriate treatments. These, of course, can be frustrating areas for a person with AIDS.

Often we assume that people know how to make decisions or recognize that they have the power to make them. This is not always true. We need to help persons with AIDS recognize their own power to make decisions—and they are faced with many. We can bring out skills to assess alternatives and consequences in evaluating the desirability of a course of action. We have to determine whether a client is having a problem in making decisions or is avoiding doing it as a result of depression or anxiety.

Signs of problems involve procrastination, denial that a decision needs to be made, rushing into an obvious option, and letting others make decisions. We have to know if the problem grows out of a lack of problem-solving skills, hopelessness, unavailable information, a sense of inadequacy or lack of freedom to choose, or interpersonal conflicts.

Active problem solving mitigates the dependent and passive patient role and increases one's cognitive, verbal, and behavioral self-assertion. Going through a decision-making process helps one to adapt. There is psychological preparation, the appropriate "work of worrying"; one feels more in control, and hence less helpless, resentful, and regretful. People who are active in making decisions about their treatment and their lives at this crucial point are more compliant about medical treatments and have fewer difficulties with the side effects of those treatments, which they have helped to choose.

In general, health-related stressors bring out more emotion-focused coping and less problem-focused coping. Weisman, Worden, and Sobel (1980) found that less problem-focused coping and fewer family resources are important predictors of depressive symptoms in people with cancer. We all need to teach and encourage problem-focused coping strategies—including encouraging and helping people to find information and obtain medical care. We can encourage them to maintain or develop physical, work, volunteer, and political activities.

Coping Strategies

One of the prime ways to increase coping ability is through social support, with communication an essential ingredient. Facilitating communication involves the giving and sharing of information, the expression of feelings, and the maintenance of self-esteem and dignity as a battle against depersonalization.

One problem of persons with AIDS that makes coping more difficult is the social stigma attached to the disease. Often persons with AIDS are not afforded the concern, caring, and empathy usually given those who have a life-threatening illness because social homophobia leads people to blame the victims. If we can believe that people suffer because they did something wrong or are guilty we can feel protected. If somehow the person with AIDS or with cancer can be seen as responsible for his illness, then fear that the same fate may befall us will be allayed. As illogical as it is, this is a way of trying to make sense out of a senseless experience, one way of warding off some of our own fears about having a life-threatening illness.

If a person with AIDS internalizes the "blame" for his illness, feelings of inferiority, inadequacy, and rejection are easily aroused and can seriously impair the ability to cope. Often, based on previous experience, the expectation of hostility arouses anger or a sense of guilt. In our study, we found that the more positive a person is about disclosing his homosexuality to others, the less likely he is to use avoidance and isolation as a coping strategy, the less angry he feels and less anxious he is as well. A positive attitude about one's homosexuality results in less

Table 9.1. Current Concerns of Persons with AIDS

	AIDS (N=46)	Cancer (N=59)
Existence	.63	.66
Work/Finances	.48	.42
Self-esteem	.41	.53
Friendship	.34	.31
Health	.22	.34
Religion	.18	.36

mood disturbance, depression, and fatigue (Wolcott, Namir et al. in press). Encouraging that positive attitude toward oneself helps to counter the stress on all coping strategies.

We also found that the most pressing concerns of persons with AIDS are related to existential issues. These include concerns about the future, the length of one's life, the quality of that life. Second in importance are concerns about work and finances; third and fourth are concerns about one's self-esteem and one's friends and social existence, including being lonely, having to move, needing to ask for assistance, social isolation, sexual dissatisfaction, blaming oneself, feeling irritable, guilty, and moody. Only after these four concerns came health concerns.

These findings are similar to those about persons with cancer, although they have more health and family concerns than persons with AIDS. (See table 9.1.) The concerns are correlated with social support and coping strategies. Those who have close friends and others to help in times of need have less of a mood disturbance, including depression. (See table 9.2.) They also have greater self-esteem and lower levels of other concerns. Persons who use avoidance coping experience more concerns than those who use an active behavioral or an active cognitive coping style. Furthermore, persons who use avoidance experience greater distress, depression, and lower self-esteem. (See table 9.3.)

Clearly, use of avoidance coping, whose goal is to avoid having to face some of the fears and anxieties and depressions of having AIDS, is not working. It is not protecting people from these distressful feelings and concerns. The higher the self-esteem, the fewer concerns people had and the better their mood states were. Therefore, I feel that inter-

Table 9.2. Correlations Among Support Network, Mood Disturbance, Concerns, and Self-Esteem

	Close friends	People to help	Satisfaction Amount	Satisfaction Emotional
TMD(+)	−.34*	−.34*	−.54***	−.57***
Depression	−.26	−.35*	−.52***	−.54***
Anxiety	−.11	−.23	−.46**	−.57***
Anger	−.25	−.28	−.40**	−.52**
Self-esteem	−.35*	−.26	−.50***	−.57***
Total concerns	−.11	−.21	−.53***	−.46**

*P < .05
**P < .01
***P < .001
(+) total mood disturbance

Table 9.3. Correlations Among Coping Strategies, Mood States, and Self-Esteem

	Active-Behavioral	Active-Cognitive	Avoidance
TMD(+)	−.45**	−.16	.27
Depression	−.31*	−.05	.43**
Anxiety	−.22	−.06	.31*
Self-esteem	.36*	.23	.47**

*P < .05
**P < .01
(+) total mood disturbance

ventions need to focus on coping abilities, protection and enhancement of self-esteem, an *active* approach to problem solving and the provision and maintenance of emotional support. (See table 9.4.)

More specifically, participants in our study who were better psychologically were using an active form of coping called positive involvement. This includes taking vitamins, maintaining a healthful diet, de-

Table 9.4. Correlations Between Concerns and Coping Strategies

Concerns	Avoidance	Active-Behavioral	Active Cognitive
Health	.37*	.07	.23
Existence	.42**	−.34*	−.10
Friends	.50***	−.28	.17
Self	.44**	.16	.14
Total	.44**	−.19	.21

*P < .05
**P < .01
***P < .001

veloping themselves as people, being involved in political activities related to AIDS, and enjoying everyday things more than previously.

Distraction also proved a successful coping strategy, in terms of mood disturbance. This includes going out more socially, relying on friends, treating oneself in special ways—activities that prevent obsessing about the illness. Those who presented the highest level of mood disturbance were engaged in solitary and passive behaviors, including cognitive ruminations about better times and how they could have done things differently.

On the whole, although persons with AIDS have small networks, ranging from six to seven others whom they consider close to them (Namir et al. n.d.), they are generally satisfied with the quality of that support. Their needs are mostly for emotional support and illness-related support. In addition, one area with which they were dissatisfied is the amount of physical contact as expression of concern and caring. I think we all have to help to bridge that gap as well—to help them feel that they are not isolated and they are getting the human contact that is so critical for their mental health. (See table 9.5.)

Group interventions are a popular and cost-effective way to intervene with persons with AIDS. I think, however, that more attention needs to be paid to the types of interventions planned in these groups. At UCLA we conducted a study of different types of group interventions—including education and relaxation training, problem-solving groups, and emotional support groups. Group participants and group leaders evaluated each session. The relaxation/education component

Table 9.5. Social Support Needs and Satisfaction

Type of support	Very important %	Very satisfied %
Emotional	68	63
Illness-related emotional	58	55
Specific	58	68
Advice	50	60
Socializing	28	53
Praise/criticism	25	55
Physical contact	25	34
Chores/tasks	5	29

was very well received, and people found the activities extremely helpful. The problem-solving group was found helpful in teaching new skills and dealing with specific problems in a structured way. The emotional support group appeared to have the most problems, with people commenting that the *lack* of structure was anxiety-producing, and that they had a need for more specific information and skills and for less participant complaint.

We found that those who participated in groups are using less avoidance coping and more active coping at our "Time 2" data collection than they had at "Time 1," whereas those who did not participate were using avoidance slightly more at "Time 2."

It is clear from our research that individuals who actively engage in attempting to cope with the illness fare better than individuals who do not. This is consistent with the literature that has found a "fighting spirit" to be associated with survival. Being oversolicitous toward a sick person can make him feel impaired. The importance of self-esteem and its association with positive measures means that strategies that focus on encouraging and building self-esteem will increase feelings of control and combat despairing helplessness.

I want to mention briefly the concerns about mental health practitioners who have clients with AIDS. The demands are great. As we are all sadly aware, more and more people are being diagnosed with ARC and AIDS, and fewer and fewer people are coming forward to work with them. One has to be especially well informed and capable of working with all other disciplines in a cooperative and collaborative way to ensure continuity and coordination of care. Often we are called on as therapists, psychologists, social workers, nurses to demystify medical issues, and to be the contact person who can be reached more easily to answer questions and respond to daily concerns.

This work demands a high degree of support, optimism, and flexibility. Being resourceful and practical helps. Not letting our own feelings of helplessness and despair interfere is crucial—especially when we are going through repetitive grief reactions. It is easy to become defensive, to protect ourselves from identification with clients who are very ill or dying, and to create distance from their pain and their anger. We need actively to seek support and/or treatment for ourselves to prevent burnout and help us to continue to provide care in a nondefensive and intensive way for those we seek to help.

In conclusion, I urge mental health practitioners who have clients with AIDS to maintain close contact with clients' physicians, know what medications are being taken and how they may affect clients' functioning; focus on enhancing coping abilities, rather than "uncovering" or insight therapy; work toward protection and enhancement of self-esteem; and encourage flexibility, optimism, and a practical style of problem solving.

References

Namir, S., M. J. Alumbaugh, F. I. Fawzy, and D. L. Wolcott. n.d. Acquired immune deficiency syndrome and social support. University of California, Los Angeles-NPI, Department of Psychiatry. Typescript.

Weisman, A. D., J. W. Worden, and H. J. Sobel. 1980. *Psychosocial screening and intervention with cancer patients.* Washington, D.C.: National Cancer Institute. Research report No. 19797.

Wolcott, D. L., F. I. Fawzy, J. Landsverk, and M. McCombs. In press. Psychosocial service needs and community organization service utilization of "AIDS-affected" individuals. *J of Psychosoc Onc.*

Wolcott, D. L., S. Namir, F. I. Fawzy, M. S. Gottlieb, and R. T. Mitsuyasu. In press. Illness concerns, attitudes toward homosexuality, and social support in gay men with AIDS. *Gen Hosp Psychiatry.*

10

Impact of Risk Reduction on Mental Health

JOHN R. ACEVEDO

Reducing the risks of contracting AIDS has an impact on mental health that can be understood by means of the clinical models that have been developed by the AIDS Health Project in the course of its work. The AIDS Health Project, sponsored by the University of California, San Francisco, and the San Francisco Department of Public Health, originally worked with gay and bisexual men only.

Identifying At-Risk Populations

By definition, risk reduction applies only to individuals who do not have the disease in question—in this case, AIDS. The course of the AIDS epidemic brought shifts in the at-risk population, and in 1985, we witnessed increased incidences among intravenous drug users and sexual partners of people at risk, particularly women. The AIDS Health Project also identified a group of resistant clients, primarily gay men, who were unable to change at-risk sexual behaviors.

The extraordinary health crisis has generated many psychodynamic issues for clients. In all populations, individuals with underlying personality and characterological disorders were identified. Included in this presentation will be the discussion of appropriate treatment strategies for both individual and group settings.

For purposes of surveillance, there is a uniform medical definition of AIDS from the Centers for Disease Control (CDC). Of the groups assigned by CDC, persons with AIDS comprise the smallest group. The next category in size of population, ARC, does not have a uniform definition. The AIDS Health Project has defined ARC as medical conditions indicative of a suppressed immune system, presenting with a full range of symptoms, but not meeting the case definition of AIDS.

The symptoms have been divided between two categories: mild-to-moderate and severe.

Mild-to-moderate symptoms include night fever, chills, sweats, weight loss, loss of appetite, fatigue, and sometimes loss of sex drive. Infections—the full range: viral, fungal, bacterial, and protozoan—are also included in this grouping. The key feature of mild-to-moderate ARC infections, however, is responsiveness to medication. In most cases, the body is able to utilize medication to fight off the infection. In addition, individuals in this category are usually employable, although sporadic periods of fatigue represent problems for employment and social interaction.

The severe ARC category presents with the same symptomology and the same range of infections. The key feature, however, is the persistent and recurrent quality of the infections. Profound fatigue and severity of infections inhibit individuals from employment and social interaction. Medical disability status is the norm in this group.

Although two discrete groups can be described, clients often present with confusion and ambivalence about the categories. The intake process includes (1) a medical history, (2) a sexually transmitted disease history, and (3) a history of therapy experiences. It also (4) allows clients to define their own illness.

A word about indications of central nervous system disorders. Particular note is made when clients describe histories of headaches, dizzy spells, visual or auditory complaints, short-term memory loss, or recent unusual behavioral changes. Neurological follow-up can be recommended for unusual complaints.

The last and largest category is the "Worried Well," for lack of better terminology. The clients in this category are asymptomatic upon presentation. Some report isolated incidences of infection that exacerbate levels of fear, anxiety, and guilt. Persons with positive antibody tests often experience confusion about their status. Are they Worried Well or do they have ARC? We encourage individuals with positive antibody test results and no other medical conditions to think of themselves as Worried Well. Once other medical conditions develop, we usually consider them in the ARC category. These clients experience the same ranges of reactions.

Women present in both categories, ARC and Worried Well. It is important not to discount fears of transmission and contagion. Issues of confidentiality are presented, and women clients need to be guaranteed the same privacy as all other clients.

Descriptions of Target Populations

Beginning with the Worried Well category, we find among clients a great need for information. Referrals to appropriate resource agencies, medical journals, and community individuals help some clients. Many clients in this category express strong psychological needs. It is important to maintain an overview of this health crisis because the bottom line is death.

Denial may present in some individuals as a cavalier attitude. Increases in sexual activity and substance abuse are characteristic of AIDS-related denial. But social and sexual withdrawal is observed in other individuals in this group. Although fear of exposure motivates some clients to be reclusive and reject potential supports, this category also presents with a deep need for support—medical, social, and emotional. Support groups provide emotional and social validation and in some cases an opportunity for sharing medical information.

The next category, ARC, exhibits a range similar to that of the Worried Well. The intensity described by clients is, however, remarkable. Of note is the powerful element of uncertainty. The lack of information about ARC and its treatment increases clients' psychological, emotional, and social needs. Clients report shock, anger, fear, sadness, and depression—with few resources or supports to assist with the coping process. The issue of uncertainty for some clients manifests in physiological reactions: an exhausting, hypertense state of awareness.

Loss issues abound in the ARC category in regard to many aspects of life: physical status, self-esteem, sexuality, relationships and other social supports, and financial support. Clients in the ARC category have the most need for support, for validation of their experiences, both physiological and psychological. Unfortunately, this is the one population that has slipped through government service gaps.

Clinical Aspects of At-Risk Populations

From work with AIDS Health Project clients, clinical models have been developed to help mental health practitioners understand better the issues presented in these categories. From attitudes of withholding to those of disclosure we find a continuum. Withholding has two aspects: protection and denial. On one hand, clients withhold information either to protect themselves or others or to deny that disease exists. Disclosure, on the other hand, can increase intimacy and trust, when information is shared, or it can bring about increased vulnerability.

This model of the continuum provides structure and a context for understanding conflicting feelings. It is also used to reinforce clients' previously developed skills around disclosure of sexual preference or experiences. Clients are encouraged to see a parallel between "coming out" as a sexual person and "coming out" with AIDS/ARC issues.

Clients are asked, for example, to think about an initial sexual experience. Who was told about that experience and what was told to them? Such discussions elicit additional issues. This model allows clients to give validation to the feelings they experience and to talk about them.

The decision for disclosure is not based solely on feelings of independence versus those of dependence. The client's *perceived* sense of these variables, however, is important. The object is to *empower* the client. Reframing the disclosure decision into the question "What can I do to feel more in control?" helps the client define for himself the boundaries for independence, structure, and the like.

Merging as an attitude has dual qualities. Some clients experience merging in a positive way—getting closer to friends, family, and community—as identification and validation. Solidarity is experienced. For others, merging represents a confrontation with reality. There is a negative identification and validation. One client stated, "Now I know I'm an ARC, and there is no turning back." This client felt more in control by declining a support group.

Complaining assists clients to develop a context for behavior changes, to discern differences between real and imagined or anticipated problems.

Our experience in using these models reinforces the notion that professionals need to take a more active educational role in dealing with AIDS-related issues. Providers who present a blank therapeutic screen for clients may only exacerbate problems.

One area that must always be addressed is the issue of homophobia, and mental health practitioners stress it. Male homophobia will be the focus because, statistically, gay men comprise the largest group affected by AIDS. When one grows up in a homophobic society, negative thoughts and feelings have a way of becoming internalized. How many people can remember their parents saying, "Gee, gay men really are nice. Let's invite those neighbor boys over for dinner." No, we grew up with exactly the opposite message. And for many gay men, in spite of all the advances of the gay movement, negative messages have resurfaced with AIDS. Some clients say, "Maybe Mom and Dad were right," or "Perhaps the church was right."

By examining the historical context, we may better understand this conflict. Before the sexual revolution in the 1960s, gay men were not openly encouraged to express their identity or to experiment sexually. Utilizing Stonewall, in 1969, as the point from which the gay movement achieved visible momentum, gay men were encouraged to express openly their sexual identity, to "come out." Stonewall was a gay bar in New York City where, in a raid by the police, customers resisted. It is significant because gay individuals fought back, expressing their right to civil liberties, for the first time.

From this point on gay men were encouraged to be proud, to express their sexual identity. For many men in the era of the sexual revolution this meant to be sexual—to have as much sex and with as many partners as possible, whenever possible. In fact, for some men liberation was measured quantitatively. AIDS has had a harrowing effect on that sense of identity.

This phenomenon can be described conceptually. Personal identity and sexual identity are not static in relation to each other but merge and disassociate at different times. Personal identity includes all of one's strengths and weaknesses. Conscious sexual identity is portrayed as developmental. Thus, for a child, sexual identity is separated from personal identity. As cognition of sexual identity develops, sexual identity moves closer toward merging with the personal identity. Movement is affected, of course, by external variables, that is, familial, cultural, political, geographical influences. For many gay men, sexual identity was limited to sexual activities/behaviors, and this notion was reinforced by the prevailing sexual mores and the gay movement.

For such gay men, moving to a major urban area represented an opportunity for the merging of personal and sexual identities. During the 1970s, gay sexual freedom flourished. With the advent of AIDS and the necessity for changes in sexual behavior came an apparent identity crisis. Clients state, "How can I be gay if I can't do the things I used to?"

It is important to acknowledge and validate this experience of loss. Not only are clients dealing with the death and loss of community members but also are faced with the loss of sexual activities and the existential loss of identity. An appropriate parallel is the female client's identity crisis upon mastectomy and hysterectomy. Each has the right to mourn and grieve. The grieving process may include anger, especially anger toward other gay men. With the invisible enemy that AIDS is, the opportunity arises to focus on internalized homophobia—the blaming of gay men for AIDS.

On the surface are behavior changes in general, eliciting feelings of fear, frustration, anger, and sadness. Clients become aware, through these feelings, of homophobia, illness, and loss. On a deeper existential level, death, love and/or lovers, and the meaning of life are confronted.

Intervention Strategies

Clients are encouraged to become aware of feelings generated by these issues and to understand the range of reactions available. Feelings are acknowledged and validated; and the grief process provides a context. Problem solving, behavioral changes, and the development of new meanings are directions for the client to approach when ready.

Death and loss are the bottom line. Death elicits major power and control issues. In addition, gay men are socialized and conditioned as men. They are taught to be in control, to know what to do, and not to be afraid, just like nongay men. Clients are encouraged to view the gamut of possible reactions as a model for developing responses that help them feel more in control and better about themselves. In addition, we introduce the concept of a warm, nurturing gay parent. We suggest the creation of that kind of internal gay parent who, like all parents, has the ability to set limits in a loving way.

An educational approach to health has proved valuable. The AIDS Health Project developed a multidimensional approach, which takes into consideration a wide range of variables (and allows for increased client self-determination), thus differing from a traditional medical model of health as the absence of disease.

The variables, of equal importance, are easily identified—thought, feelings, physiology, environment, spirituality, social supports, behavior. I would like to elaborate on three. The first two are thoughts and feelings. For our purposes, we define feelings as immediate emotional reactions, and thoughts as sentences I tell myself. Negative, destructive, and unnecessary thoughts contribute, of course, to feeling out of control and to attitudes of hopelessness and helplessness. Utilizing cognitive techniques, we teach skills to redirect thought patterns into more positive, constructive, and necessary modes. These thoughts contribute to a sense of control and attitudes of hopefulness and responsibility. The latter attitude is reframed into the ability to respond to a particular situation.

In regard to spirituality, another variable in our multidimensional approach to health, I found that many gay men have rejected a formal religious structure or organization, but they have retained their own values or belief systems. By acknowledging and validating spirituality, we hold the door open for exploration and development. The health crisis has motivated many gay men to return to religion, only to find that it does not completely address their needs. Developing new meanings of spirituality as a reaction to health issues reinforces client self-determination and control.

Group Treatment

Initially, the AIDS Health Project's Worried Well and ARC educational groups were composed primarily of Caucasian males (83.5 percent), ranging in age from twenty to fifty-seven. Group members tended to be well educated and employed (50 percent). Forty percent said that they lived alone, and the mean length of residence in the Bay Area was ten years. The AIDS Health Project began actively recruiting Third World group members and facilitators in 1985 with one Third World group then in process. Addressing cross-cultural issues remains the biggest challenge for all AIDS-related agencies. The groups, which are closed, meet for eight weeks, once a week for two hours. Each member is screened to assure maximum service provision. A fee of twenty or forty dollars is requested for any Worried Well group, and no one is turned away for lack of funds. There are three groups for the Worried Well: Stress Reduction, Hot and Healthy Sex, and Integrated Health—a comprehensive group. There are two ARC groups: Mild-to-Moderate and Severe. An educational support model is followed. We are teaching skills to cope with the health crisis and to make behavioral changes—all in the context of a supportive environment. This is not a therapy group, but whenever AIDS, sex, and death are addressed, intense feelings may arise.

The groups are led by trained facilitators who are able to redirect discussion back to the educational model when necessary. The educational model provides a structure to contain feelings as well as a role model for teaching self-containment skills. The group context also provides a place for generating ideas in terms of developing the ability to respond to the health crisis. Group leaders are always available for brief meetings and crisis sessions and especially for referrals to other city resources and private therapists. Groups are an excellent adjunct to therapy; nevertheless, clients are told that groups do not take the place of therapy.

Individuals who are psychotic, suicidal, or currently abusing alcohol or drugs are inappropriate for the Worried Well/ARC groups. They are referred to more appropriate resources. Also, the issues and models presented here are applicable for use within individual sessions. Practitioners, however, need to feel comfortable with an educational role in a situation requiring flexibility.

In conclusion, the psychosocial issues associated with AIDS-related risk reduction are multifaceted and complex. The importance of a thorough assessment cannot be emphasized enough. Preexisting psychiatric disorder must be addressed. Both individual and group models are appropriate for assisting clients in their response to AIDS, for developing more appropriate coping skills, and for changing at-risk behaviors. Practitioners need to appreciate how different sexual identities and personality organizations may affect the individual responses to AIDS. The psychoeducational group model utilized by the AIDS Health Project includes strengthening client support systems and coping skills, while teaching specific skills and techniques to manage stress, depression, anger, and the uncertainty of the illness.

11

Counseling HIV Seropositives

MARK GOLD, NEIL SEYMOUR, JEFFREY SAHL

The antibody test for HIV was developed by Robert Gallo and his associates at the National Institutes of Health in Bethesda, Maryland. Originally devised to screen blood for antibodies to HIV, the test has been successful. With the psychosocial interview, the hepatitis test, and now the AIDS antibody test, the chances of a person—even a hemophiliac, for whom blood is now heat-treated—being infected with the virus through a blood transfusion are small.

The alternative test site program was developed because health departments were concerned that people would donate blood at blood banks, where it was tested, and request the test results. Even though there is a very low false-positive, false-negative rate, there was concern that instead of protecting the blood supply, the false negatives would in fact work in reverse and endanger it. Therefore, in most states, one can be tested for the antibody and obtain test results at an alternative site under specific programs. The alternative sites include special medical centers, research projects, private physicians, and clinics.

Populations To Be Tested

The critical question arises of who should take this test: those persons who have some reason to believe that they have been infected, those in a high-risk group—gay and bisexual men, anyone who shares needles (hemophiliacs are mostly tested through hospital hematology departments), and partners of people who are at risk.

Many people want to take the test. A classic example is a man who visited a prostitute seven years ago, once, and is now worried that he has AIDS. How to handle people like that, to reassure them about a casual contact—a point that comes up repeatedly—is important in screening. If people want to know whether they are infectious, if they want information that can reinforce safe behavior, if they want to know whether they have been infected through sexual contact, needles, or transfusions, or if people at risk are considering pregnancy or initiating new gay relationships, they should consider taking the test.

Before people take the test, we ask them to think about the difference between *assuming* that they are positive and *knowing* that they are positive. On one hand, if a person makes the assumption, because he or she has been involved in risky behavior, that he or she is positive, then perhaps that person does not need to take the test, which can be a traumatic experience. On the other hand, some people are engaged in compulsive sexual behavior, and for them taking the test can be a sort of confrontation. Being told in fact, "Yes, you are positive," has helped a number of people to make behavioral changes.

Those who have lovers diagnosed with AIDS or ARC naturally wonder about their own status. Others desire to know their status in anticipation of future possible required nonanonymous testing—military or employment screenings, for example. Some desire information before making major life decisions. Finally, there are those who want to confirm a previous test result.

In pretest groups we notice that people do not know what to expect the test to answer, and they want it to answer things it cannot answer, specifically, "Will I get AIDS?" "Will I live a long life?" "Will I live a happy life?" We cannot stress enough that the test will not tell if one is going to die of AIDS. Nor could any counseling give definitive answers about one's longevity or well-being.

Pretest Education in San Francisco

Availability of the test is advertised in local newspapers. People in San Francisco are encouraged to call the AIDS Foundation Hotline for more information about the test to help them decide whether or not it is appropriate for them. If they decide to come in for more information, they make an appointment through the phone bank. In groups of four to seven or eight people, they see a ten-minute videotape that describes the test in greater detail. In a group discussion they can ask questions of the health educator, or they can speak privately with the health educator if they have specific questions that embarrass them. Frequently, the health educator will call on the counselors to meet individually with people who are having difficulty with the decision.

If they still want to have their blood tested, in another area their blood is drawn, and a return appointment is made for two weeks later.

No names are given at any point. When people call the phone bank for their first appointment, they make up their own code number of two letters and two numbers. Upon arriving for that initial appointment, they simply use those numbers and letters. They are then assigned a number that goes on their tube of blood and is used for the return appointment.

People are given a list of resources for the two-week waiting period, which, for many, is a very difficult time. Upon returning, they meet with a counselor privately. Again, only the number is exchanged—no names are used. At that point the result is given. People are helped to understand the test result, and appropriate referrals are made to resources in the community. A follow-up videotape and resource list are also given. At the end of the session we offer to those who are seropositive or seronegative the opportunity to see a follow-up counselor for a free hour consultation to consider questions or help with problems in adjustment. Few people find this extra session necessary.

Counseling

A four-day training is required of counselors at the San Francisco AIDS Foundation who give out test results. Dr. Constance Wofsy of San Francisco General Hospital and UC San Francisco gives an introductory course on AIDS. A woman from the Women's Aware Study talks about issues of women and AIDS. (See chapter by Shaw and Paleo below.) A psychologist talks about issues for gay men, as do an epidemiologist and a counselor. Role-playing giving a positive result, role-playing receiving a positive or a negative result, and getting constructive feedback are helpful for trainers. Anonymity is distinguished from confidentiality, and how to give results to someone whose name you don't know is taught. (Basically, use the word "you.") Some test recipients give their names; most do not.

Intervention has three goals. The first is to help the person absorb the news and cope with the results, to be able to walk out on the street again. The second is to connect the person to resources. No matter how good the counseling, many do not really hear much of what goes on because they are in shock. Even with negative results, the situation is very complicated. If someone is all geared up for a positive test result, and gets a negative, his or her whole world is turned upside down. When one is prepared to die, or prepared to have this thing hanging over one's head, a negative test result is not just a reprieve. Finally, the third is to counsel people as much as possible about health education: risk reduction, safe sex, how to stay healthy and asymptomatic and, most importantly, how to reduce or eliminate the possibility of infecting others. We rely very much on the guidelines for AIDS risk reduction that were developed by the San Francisco AIDS Foundation, and people walk out with several packets.

Each counselor has a checklist. We confirm and reconfirm the person's code number to avoid any mix-up. Giving the results is divided into four parts: establishing rapport quickly with the person; giving results as clearly and straightforwardly as possible; working on emotional and cognitive integration, the heart of the interview; and finally, developing a plan. We cannot promise simple behavioral solutions to somebody because the research data simply do not support them, despite our hopes. For now we try to give a sense of some control and instill better health habits.

We talk about alcohol and drugs, further infection, not spreading it to others, the possible need for further resources, its personal meaning, and telling other people, such as physicians or lovers.

Informing others is a big issue. We discuss with the person whom to tell, whom not to tell, how to tell them, what that would be like. Telling a lover could result in violent conflict, perhaps a breakup, or it could make the two feel closer. That subject alone could require about ten hours of counseling, so much is involved.

We make sure that at least the person walks out with a resource list and a referral to a counselor. Most people will have a delayed reaction. People are often numb, which is why that resource list is so critical.

We have a plan for potential suicides. We are in touch with the emergency rooms and psychiatric units. It's much more likely, however, that any kind of an emergency reaction will be subacute, necessitating only a walk-in clinic. Here are a few issues that come up during the counseling sessions: substance abuse, fear of sex or sex-phobias (many people report being celibate), sexual addiction, sexual identity problems, relationship conflicts, grief over loss or anticipated loss of friends or lovers, general health concerns, excessive anxiety or hypochondriasis or extreme anxiety responses, whom and how to tell, coming out, quality of life, continuing risky behaviors, unwillingness to change sexual behaviors, unwillingness to alter behaviors around cofactors (such as drug use or nutrition), stress reduction, establishing and utilizing a support network, fears of intimacy, health education, health planning, transmission, parenting, and fear of illness or death. There's an awful lot to deal with in a half-hour to an hour.

Use of Groups for Post-Test Education and Counseling

Since September 1985, we have led groups for more than 200 men, all gay white males. We started the testing on July 1, 1985, and the groups started soon after. The time frame from knowing the results to group participation has ranged from one day to more than three months. The format of the group is first of all informational, allowing questions as a form of building rapport, and second, a supportive group process with an issue focus. The issues are self-defined and amazingly consistent over time. The groups are an hour and a half long and each session is open to new members. The mean attendance for the men is just under two group sessions.

Confidentiality has never seemed to be a problem. People give their first names only. The major concern first voiced in these groups is the method of obtaining results. It is a credit to the Department of Public Health that people generally have been very pleased about how they received the results in San Francisco. It's an easy way to get warmed up, "How did you find out, when did you find out?" These people come to group therapy voluntarily and probably are a little more upset than most. They vividly report an experience of the *mood* in which test results were given. They recall the feeling of the counselor and specifically they appreciate not having received the results at the beginning of the interview.

In settings other than the alternative sites, people receive the results in brief telephone calls from, for example, a health worker. We have heard some fairly bad stories, such as getting positive results from doctor's offices, and then at the time of the next physical examination noting the doctors and nurses putting on gloves. Right after giving results that just does not work. People feel pretty bad anyway. In the initial feedback session when one gets results, a supportive session is most helpful, although very little information can be imparted at this point.

Group members have reported a progression of psychological reactions over time. Days one to three constitute a kind of psychological shock. The first emotion that people report is anger rather than denial: anger at the medical community, anger at the government, anger at various agents, often a projection—questions like "Who did this to me?" "Why did I do this to myself?" Many express problems with their religious beliefs at this time. More than one person asked how God could allow this to happen to them. There is also free-floating anger, leading to suicidal and homicidal thinking, some individuals expressing feelings of wanting to drive into people in the street, for example. The first three days then are a critical time for supportive services.

From three days to three months there are waves of depression, with accompanying sleep, eating, and mood disturbances, a sense of isolation and alienation, as well as impotence and a decrease in libidinal drives. Many body image questions come up—feelings of being diseased, feelings of being impotent in the face of this disease, and feelings of being contagious. Sex in a way becomes deadly, sex becomes evil. Self-image can suffer from this alienation. Some report walking down the street feeling dirty, feeling different. Meeting with other people who are seropositive helps a great deal during this time.

Awareness of being seropositive for HIV can promote a sense of weakness of the body, of the self. The knowledge that antibodies cannot fight off the virus, in fact, leads to a certain sense of a weakening of the self, into which the whole question of the will enters, a fundamental kind of psychological problem. Since one cannot do anything, one feels hopeless and impotent. In psychological terms, a positive HIV result can lead to a breaking down of the defense structure. We have a defense structure that's good and that protects us. In the face of death, disease, and disfigurement, we can erect a certain level of denial. The seropositive result fairly effectively shatters that denial, along with other defenses. This can lead to suicidal ideation, decompensation, depersonalization.

With the decline of the defenses, death comes right up to one's face. It can be a very important time to make life changes, but a very supportive environment is needed to do that. Thus, the leader of groups for seropositive individuals needs an understanding of these existential issues.

Psychodynamically, inadequacy, nurturance, and trust themes emerge, the nurturance and trust themes coming from a sense of being affected by the nurturing object. In this case, the nurturing object of sexual affection leads to a disease; in HIV transmission, the person who has it becomes that diseased object and passes it on. That is why a very supportive, nurturing environment is essential to encourage the development of new defenses. Denial is one of the biggest defenses to shatter, and it is fairly primitive. Effective leaders may suggest higher level defenses, such as intellectualization or rationalization, as a means of coping, and let the group work it through, using as much information as members can absorb at a given moment.

We encourage people not to talk to others outside the group about their test results for a while, until those defenses come back and are a little stronger. Participants have related stories about their experiences, for example, longtime roommates who have moved out, one physician telling a man that he should not live with his children whom he then shipped away to his mother's house. We tell people to live with the results for a while themselves, adjust to it, until they are ready to deal with others.

This is also a great time to encourage self-exploration. We use the short follow-up group to investigate problem identification, for example: A man comes in who is seropositive. He says the next thing he wants to do is get a helper/suppressor-cell ratio test. Why does he want to get this T-cell count? He says because he likes to drink a little. He presents his denial: "You know, I'm seropositive, but if my T-cells are all right, it's probably okay that I go ahead and drink a little more. But if it's bad, if my immune system's gone, then maybe I'll stop drinking." You can do a little mild confrontation here, identifying the problem for the person in a very supportive way, and perhaps send him on his way to a substance abuse program.

People are very anxious to hang onto anything you can offer, like a plan to protect their health. Legal plans also come up a lot. People have concerns about what will happen when they die—they equate seropositivity with dying. Psychological advice of the very simplest kind is well taken. Sex is often a question, and along with this of course the emotional release that people need. Most people just lose their sex drive for a while, and for some people that becomes a focal issue and they need to go to a safe sex group or a "hot and healthy" sex group.

Rephrasing the situation into a positive experience is immensely helpful. The positive HIV result is useful for carrying on one's life, facing up to major existential questions. This result can bring a certain immanence to life. It may be time for bibliotherapy—to go back and read that old philosophy that didn't make too much sense when you were in college but may make a lot of sense now, about what it means to be alive today.

People who are seropositive are a new group. Potentially, they might live the rest of their lives being contagious, carrying a disease that can kill other people, and yet they might also live fully through their lives. One fellow said, "Well, I got the results, and I was thinking I want to sell my business in another city and move to San Francisco. There are people like me here and it's supportive here, and when I get sick, or if I get sick, there'll be care for me." The therapeutic suggestion to him was that where he lived might matter more than where he died, but if he wanted to come here and live in a supportive environment, and have fun and do whatever he wanted to do here, great. If he was coming here to die, that wasn't such a good idea. One could die anywhere.

We try to frame the basic question: Whatever the odds are for you, what can you do to improve them? How can you improve the odds of staying healthy and not passing it on? If someone doesn't ask for numbers, we don't give them, and if they ask for numbers, we talk about it and explain how tentative the statistics are. Interpretation of any new statistics about seropositivity has to consider the population base, the numbers, how the individual relates to that base, and that base as not representative of the entire population.

Conclusion

The presence of the AIDS antibody in one's blood does provoke profound questions, and the sensitive counselor can help the individual consider them in a frank, honest way. What we have found best is clear information presented in a timely fashion after the test has been performed, accompanied by appropriate referral with the added provision of supportive group experiences. AIDS has made all of us face the harder existential issues of life and death. Knowing that this confrontation is difficult and having sensitivity and compassion for those struggling with it is the basic key to good HIV antibody test counseling.

12

Mental Health Issues of Persons with AIDS

JUDY MACKS AND DAN TURNER

Sociocultural Issues That Affect Psychological Responses to AIDS

Judy Macks: The social, cultural, and political issues that surround AIDS make it a unique illness in health history. Those most at risk are regarded with varying degrees of negativity in this culture and experience many forms of discrimination. Therefore, the emotional turbulence that surrounds AIDS directly affects the person with AIDS interpersonally and intrapersonally.

The popular image of AIDS is of a white gay male disease. The image is, in fact, a myth. More than 40 percent of the people with AIDS in this country are black and Hispanic. More than a thousand women have contracted AIDS. The figures raise issues about cultural and ethnic minorities that need to be addressed in clinical practice, in addition to the issues raised by working with a largely gay and bisexual population.

Generally, gay and bisexual men and intravenous (IV) drug users as communities do not have access to significant advocacy and political power. San Francisco is noticeably unusual because its gay community does have considerable organized political power, which has led to the existence of a generous array of services for those with AIDS. Still, it remains our responsibility in part as clinicians to act as advocates for our clients, in particular for those who have few economic, political, and emotional resources. The demographics and the politics are part of what makes AIDS a unique illness.

Editor's Note: This paper approaches the issues from two perspectives: that of professional social worker Judy Macks, who has had therapeutic contact with persons with AIDS in all its phases, and that of a man with AIDS, Dan Turner, who describes his psychological process as he copes with this illness.

A consequent issue of AIDS is that we as a society, and as clinicians, must confront both our own homophobia as well as the internalized homophobia experienced by gay men. Uncovering internalized homophobia is critical to begin the process of working with a person with AIDS. A person with AIDS may experience severe guilt feelings and self-blame for contracting the illness and concomitant low self-esteem. Then, the person may feel that the illness was caused by his life-style. Questioning one's sexual orientation can be a direct result of internalized homophobia and the AIDS epidemic. Negative messages in the media as well as responses from family, friends, and employers can become internalized to varying degrees despite trying consciously to counteract such messages. To combat the frequently internalized homophobia of clients with AIDS, clinicians must emphasize that a person with AIDS is sick because he has been exposed to and has been infected by a virus.

An area of enormous sociocultural concern is that of the family, particularly in two areas. Imagine being diagnosed with a life-threatening illness, and having to tell your parents both that you may die soon and that you are gay. The decision of self-disclosure raises fear of rejection, often anxiety and panic. The experience can be devastating. I have seen a spectrum of family responses, from rallying around the person with AIDS in a consolidated support system to disowning him—total rejection.

AIDS has challenged the concept of family for many medical, mental health, and social service professionals, as they experience the gay family, often extended and nontraditional. Not all alike, gay families can include a lifelong partner, lovers, friends, children. Recognizing and respecting intimate gay relationships and granting the partner the same rights as a husband or wife with regard to medical care, involvement in the illness and in legal matters remain a challenge for professionals working with AIDS.

With AIDS, two basic aspects of people's lives are drastically altered and transformed—that of intimacy and sexuality and that of livelihood and financial situation. Since AIDS can be sexually transmitted, concerns for the partner who is also at risk for contracting AIDS arise. Feelings of contamination are common, as well as altered levels of sexual desire. Whether in a relationship or single, the questions "Is there sex after AIDS?" and "What is safe sex?" must be addressed by professionals involved in the care of persons with AIDS. The question of financial need is exacerbated by having nothing to do. For many, employment has been a source of high income, self-esteem, identity, and daily routine. Many young people with AIDS have been faced with this loss and no replacement, leaving them depressed, bored, and isolated.

Finally, the great uncertainty about AIDS and the rapidly changing ground of available and increasing medical information provoke tremendous anxiety as the person with AIDS tries to make informed choices about health care.

Dan Turner: When I was diagnosed with KS in February 1982, there were no stories or articles about AIDS in the papers. My doctor had seen only one previous case, and he could tell me only that I had a rare cardiovascular cancer, and that for some reason my immune system was not functioning properly. The acronym AIDS was not to appear in the media for six months. And by that time my cancer had already stabilized.

Before the term AIDS was used, we had the acronym GRID, or "Gay-Related Immuno-Deficiency," and the more sensational "Gay Plague." Simply the letters KS and PCP (Kaposi's sarcoma and *Pneumocystis carinii* pneumonia) were becoming familiar to the gay community.

I was a theater reviewer for the gay press and writing for the *Bay Area Reporter*. I'd been on assignment in New York in the spring of 1981, and feel that probably I was exposed to the virus at that time.

I had a subscription to the New York gay newspaper, *The New York Native*, in which two gay writers were sparring about the implications of this new threat to the gay community. Both of the writers were to write plays on the subject later. First was Larry Kramer, who reported that five of his friends had already died of KS or PCP, and he warned people in the gay community that they had better wake up and change their attitudes toward sex, or they would kill one another. He advised us to get out of the sexual olympics. He said that recreational sex was dangerous, that we were racing to our doom, and that we should get out of the fast lane. He had already written a vitriolic novel called *Faggots*, in which he attacked the urban gay life-style of drugs, disco, and one-night stands.

In contrast, Robert Chesley took issue with his moral tone and biblical-prophet stand, saying that promiscuity was not a dirty word and that gay men were expressing their sexual liberation from an oppressive, straight society. Disease was scientific. It was an inconvenience, but it should not stand in the way of our human rights. These were the articles I was reading when the first two KS lesions appeared above my right ankle in December 1981.

These arguments are still with us today: Old Testament Armageddon sanctions versus human rights. Somewhere the survival of the body and the mind can coexist. It has been our struggle to find that place.

My family knew that I was gay. Diagnosis for me was telling them that I had cancer—fear-word in itself. I chose to tell my eldest brother and his wife. They lived in California and were close enough to visit if necessary. And I might have to ask them to help me financially. I chose not to tell my mother, who lived alone in the Midwest, because she would have to worry through each examination and have no one at home to talk to. I chose not to tell my gay sister, living with her lover in rural Minnesota, because she had ulcers and was experiencing health problems of her own. I chose not to tell my born-again brother in Dallas, Texas, because I was afraid he would be judgmental and say, "I told you so," and "You should have changed your ways." Later I decided to tell him, because I figured I could use the prayers, and we were able to share the best of both worlds over the phone.

My closest housemate cried when I told him, and one friend actually fainted on the corner of 18th and Castro streets [center of a gay neighborhood]. As I caught his head before it hit the pavement, a woman rushed over and said, "Is he sick? Should I call an ambulance?" One pulled up as he revived, and I had to explain what happened. What had disturbed him was the fear that if I had the cancer he could get it, too. He knew that my life-style was moderate, that I had not used drugs or been obsessed with sex. Yet it dawned on him, as it had me, that this bug did not discriminate between the most popular guy on campus and your average Joe-gay. It was apparent that the word had to get out to the rest of the gay community, because we were all threatened by something bigger than Anita Bryant.

People with AIDS themselves and the doctors who set up the KS Clinic at the University of California, San Francisco Medical Center were the first to warn the gay community and those immediately at risk. At the time, I was earning a living word-processing at Bechtel Corporation, where Dr. Conant, from UC, had presented a slide lecture primarily on herpes, but ending with one or two slides of KS. I attended that lecture in the fall of 1981, little realizing, of course, that just a couple of months later I would have KS myself.

Bobbi Campbell, who had been diagnosed six months before I was, had started writing a column in the *Sentinel*, which informed the gay community about the problem, the testing, and the treatment that he was experiencing, and promoted his good attitude about surviving, as well as encouragement to get out of the fast lane—take care of yourself, and be good to yourself. As I began chemotherapy in March 1982 and was treated for parasites, I decided to look into alternative therapy to treat the underlying immune system disorder. I decided to have acupuncture every two weeks and learned to do active, positive visualization. I decided to be celibate until I knew how my body would fare with the treatment; getting rest and taking the sensible if cautious route were my objectives at the time.

General Psychological Issues and Responses to an AIDS Diagnosis

Judy Macks: Different stages of psychological response to an AIDS diagnosis are characterized by specific issues and tasks. The beginning stage, in which a person is diagnosed with AIDS, is a period of crisis. Emotional responses range from affective numbing to affective discharge. Often, the individual experiences shock and denial, unable to absorb information beyond learning of the diagnosis. Many people feel overwhelmed, however, and begin to be flooded with every question imaginable: whom to tell, when to tell them, treatment, family, finances, whether to go back to work. AIDS can be a long process. The therapist's task at this point is to help contain the fear and anxiety, reassuring the client that there will be time to make decisions. The sense of urgency that life is going to end today or tomorrow is an underlying fear. To help the person avoid hasty decisions that may be regretted later is vital. Anxiety often focuses on the fear of future conditions, such as becoming dependent on others and thus a burden, having visible KS lesions, losing independence and mobility, and becoming neurologically and cognitively impaired. Since many persons with AIDS have witnessed the illness and death of someone with AIDS very close to them, clients often have a realistic picture of the progression of the disease.

Suicidal ideation is commonly seen among persons with AIDS. Generally, three types of AIDS clients present with thoughts of suicide, each requiring different clinical interventions. Most common are clients who talk about it at points of crisis throughout the illness. Usually these are clients with no history of suicide responding to the diagnosis and attempting to manage feelings of despair, loss of control, helplessness, and fear of future conditions. By the time these matters come up, in fact, the person is in a very different psychological state, and the suicidal ideation has changed.

The second type is the actively suicidal AIDS client who presents with a clinical history of depression, anxiety, suicide attempts, and/or character disorder. The third type of suicidal client is the person who is very ill and considering suicide as a way to hasten the impending death. Actively suicidal AIDS clients require standard clinical interventions. I have been surprised at how low the suicide rate has been, although exact statistics on suicide related to AIDS are not available.

When clients are diagnosed, I usually use traditional crisis intervention. In terms of helping people to increase their coping abilities, remember that they have coped with other crises in the past. Because AIDS patients tend to isolate themselves when the diagnosis is made, one task is to help them reach out to those people with whom they have been intimate. Or else help them find services that can serve as lifelines for them at times of crisis.

Dan Turner: In the beginning phase, with my diagnosis of KS, I was not in pain. I had not experienced shortness of breath or loss of weight or fevers; I simply had five KS lesions above my right ankle. There was no pain, no itching. I was told that this was cancer and got the message that it might spread and kill me. I listened to the doctor's concern and felt the full impact of his words. But because I didn't feel bad physically, I decided not to pretend the disease was worse than I felt.

I chose to take this prognosis a day at a time. I had a prior health experience to fall back upon: I had learned a lesson from hepatitis. With that, I had overreacted to my feelings of exhaustion and debilitation and had psychologically convinced myself that I would not get stronger. And so for a year, I didn't get stronger, until I finally snapped out of my negative attitude. Then, and only then, did I start to feel better and feel like myself again.

Having won that personal battle five years before my diagnosis of KS, I felt I could win this new one. I knew that if I bought the negative line I would seal my fate. I had almost done it with hepatitis. This time I was prepared to fight.

In the earlier experience, doctors had told me that they could not do anything, that I would have to sit back and wait for the disease to take its course. Now, again, they were saying that there was no cure. I knew that I would have to take the responsibility for my own disease, that there was no magic bullet. I found out what the doctors could do for me, and then I looked into what I could do for myself.

I tried to go about it calmly and rationally. People around me seemed to react more emotionally, even neurotically. I could feel their personal concern and, in the case of some gay health providers, their personal fear of contracting the disease. In fact, one of them *did* contract the disease. I began to objectify my illness. I began to see it as not my problem but a problem of the gay community.

I began to externalize my personal fear. I began to lecture on my lesions. Dr. Conant took me to Stanford, where one day I explained to thirty dermatologists what KS looked like and showed them the spots on my leg. I began speaking on panels and at community forums. In May 1982, at the Harvey Milk [the assassinated gay city supervisor] birthday celebration on Castro Street, I addressed the gay community, warning them about KS and mentioning that I had run the Bay-to-Breakers race after nine chemotherapy treatments. A cheer went up and I felt supported. I felt my approach to winning had been vindicated, and my confidence grew.

I had quit my word-processing job, which had been drudge work for me, and decided to go on disability, doing only what I like to do, which was to work in the arts, specifically composing music and working in theater. Wanting to keep informed of the scientific news, I became one of the first board members of what became the San Francisco AIDS Foundation, and I continue as a board member today.

By being involved and staying informed, I felt that I was in control of the disease, it was not in control of me. My visualizations continued to be positive. I found that white sharks eating the lesions or pac-men chomping on the lesions were not strong enough images for me, so I began using some Christian imagery from my more personal religious roots. I found it deeper and more effective.

In August 1982, I was one of the first ten to begin alpha interferon trials at San Francisco General Hospital. I went off chemotherapy and began low-dose interferon, five days a week every other week. After the initial trial I continued for a year and a half, and then learned to give myself injections. Continuing with alpha interferon five days a week every third week, I have found that side effects are minimal. I do not plan to rock the boat until we have more definite data on successful treatment of AIDS, or treatment to stimulate the immune system.

I was fortunate to have had my cancer stabilized after two months of chemotherapy in April 1982. After getting rid of the parasites, I felt that my immune system was able to bounce back just enough to keep me on a relatively healthy plateau above the threshold of the immune-suppressed danger zone.

In October 1982 I met a man who became my lover for two years. He met my doctors, was physically tested himself, and was counseled about what kind of sexual activity we could share. We were intimate for more than two years and still share a friendship. His health has remained above average for a gay man. For the year and a half that we had intercourse we used condoms, which I feel was satisfactory protection.

It was wonderful to have the support of a lover during this time, and perhaps what was best about it was that I had met him *after* my diagnosis of KS, and after the media had begun using the acronym AIDS.

As the fear in the general public grew, it had its impact at home. My lover began tossing down more vitamins than I did and reacted to the news by being less sexually inclined if there had been some hysterical report that day in the paper. My housemates bought a dishwasher; one housemate began spraying the toilet seat with Lysol every time he went to the bathroom; my lover began reacting to other people with AIDS whose health he witnessed declining, and stopped taking me to the hospital for treatment. The outside world and the health of others had their impact on our private relationship.

I decided to go back to school for a master's degree in social work. I was accepted into the program at San Francisco State University and had to take a prerequisite summer course in August 1985. At the same time, my landlady raised the rent 50 percent and all my housemates moved out. I experienced some personal rejection, and stress was at an all-time high. My body finally said, "Enough is enough," and shingles broke out on my face. I spent ten days on Ward 5B, the San Francisco General Hospital AIDS ward, being treated intravenously. My right eye was still healing from the experience as I wrote this, and I have learned once more that one must plan relaxation in every day. One must actively discourage stress.

Psychological Issues and Responses During the Course of the Illness

Judy Macks: After the initial crisis resolves, AIDS patients enter a middle phase in which two distinguishing tasks emerge. The first is that of getting on with life—that is, learning to live in the face of a chronic life-threatening illness instead of waiting to die. The second task is that of facing immediate and anticipated losses, ranging from loss of mobility, independence, and self-esteem to anticipated death. Persons with AIDS, as well as those closely involved in their lives, experience the roller coaster of emotions experienced in the grief and anticipatory grief process. Ongoing tasks and processes such as life review and taking care of unfinished emotional and practical business can contribute to the ability to continue to live. This may involve attempts to resolve conflicts or resentments with loved ones and to make decisions about concrete matters such as wills, powers of attorney, and directives to physicians. Treatment failure and/or the recurrence or development of symptoms or infections can readily precipitate an emotional crisis. At this point, a client often experiences emotional exhaustion and a profound sense of hopelessness.

When a client is close to death, the focus of issues and tasks shift. Both the AIDS patient and loved ones can experience great fear of pain, abandonment, and death. Adequate pain management must be provided along with the reassurance that the client need not die in pain. Interventions must be designed to work with the entire support system by honoring the patient's wishes and facilitating the dying process for all involved.

Useful psychological interventions for persons with AIDS should encourage emotional expression, increase coping skills as much as possible, assist in managing fluctuating moods and physical states, and provide opportunities for maintaining a sense of control and mastery. Persons with AIDS request a range of treatment modalities including crisis intervention, problem-solving therapy, brief psychotherapy, supportive ongoing psychotherapy, insight-oriented psychotherapy, and/or group interventions.

Groups can be particularly useful in combating the isolation often experienced by the person with AIDS and his support system. Groups can be very fast-paced, with participants responding honestly and quickly to very deep and personal issues. Most clients have altered their sense of time; that is, knowing that they no longer have the luxury of time can help them push through to underlying issues and concerns in a way that they were not able to do before diagnosis. Structured groups that focus on cognitive and behavioral change, support, and education can be especially helpful in providing participants with a sense of control and containment for their oftentimes overwhelming emotions.

Dan Turner: In Denver, in 1983, a group of us met nationally. People with AIDS from San Francisco, New York, Houston, and Denver got together and started networking. We were attending a conference on AIDS, which had started off with people wondering what we would accomplish since there were so many different agendas.

Not until the end of the conference did persons with AIDS themselves go to the front of the room. They carried a banner that said, "Fighting for our lives." Each of us shared experiences with the entire assembly; people at the conference began to understand why they were all there. That it *was* for people with AIDS, and that it was a human issue, and we were sharing our experiences with them. I think for the first time the statistics-gathering and the note-taking were dropped, and people realized that this was a human issue and that we were dealing with life and death.

It was a very moving experience, and the keynote speaker who was to speak after us had to wait fifteen minutes until the audience dried their tears and collected themselves. We all went out to eat together—fourteen persons with AIDS at the Top of the Rockies restaurant. We were sitting at a long table, a Last Supper of sorts. At the table next to us was a wedding party—priest, family, bride, husband, and friends. Someone at our table decided, so we could all feel part of the conversation, to ask questions and go around the table, with everyone having a chance to answer. The questions started circulating: "When did you come out?" "What was your favorite sexual position?" "What did you do before you got AIDS?" "What was your female name, if you had one?"

We all got to know one another. There was one man in particular to whom I was attracted, and I began wondering if in fact I could have intimate relations with another person with AIDS. When this went through my mind, I had to ask myself a lot of the questions that I would be dealing with later when I was back out on the streets dating, or trying to date and meet people. Would people reject me? Because it would be necessary for me to tell them that I had AIDS, how would they react to me, would they run away? I had to check out my own feelings about how I would feel having sex or intimate relations with another person with AIDS.

This was a slow process for me, but I was able to do that, and to feel comfortable about it. Last year I met a friend whose lover was diagnosed with KS. When the dermatologist told him, the guy asked, "Well, what do I do now?" The doctor told him, "Some people do chemotherapy, some people do vitamins." So, he was rather left on his own, and the guy decided that he didn't want to try chemotherapy. He went to a vitamin shop, stocked up, and was trying to help himself that way. My friend called me and said, "I want you to come over and talk to my lover about what you've done."

I went there for dinner and I was concerned because I felt that the guy was developing symptoms for pneumocystis. He was coughing and he was short of breath. So I encouraged him to go to San Francisco General Hospital to be monitored by doctors there. Eventually, he did go and we became close friends. What I discovered is that people with AIDS hang on to their personalities, who they really are, even though they are threatened with death. In fact, they hang on to their personalities even more tenaciously.

This particular person was a gentleman and a charming man. We traveled up the coast together and spent a lot of time together. I felt that he would survive. I felt that his KS was minimal and that, like myself, he would make it.

Well, his situation deteriorated. He did, in the spring, develop *Pneumocystis carinii* pneumonia. Then, when he was in the hospital recuperating, he developed some type of brain infection and the doctors wanted to do a brain biopsy. Mark decided against that.

He went home, where he tried to recuperate. He'd have good days and bad days, and his friends rallied around him. I spent time with him. He started having seizures, which eventually got worse. I could see him trying to hang on; being the gentleman that he was, he wanted to take me to lunch—I had been taking him lunch—and on a good day he called me up and said, "I want to take you to lunch."

So he did. Then eventually he was planning a trip back to Boston to be with his family, and his lover was to follow. He did go back to Boston and he died there.

One day I remember he looked at me and he said that he was jealous of my health. He said he did not understand why I was surviving and he could not. He tried very hard, and I think what is so remarkable about him was how he was able to keep his sense of dignity throughout.

Death and Dying and Countertransference Issues

Judy Macks: Clinicians experience, along with their AIDS clients, the emotions of the grieving process. The key to successful clinical work with AIDS patients lies in our willingness to look at our own attitudes and fears about death and dying. The feelings of helplessness, loss of control, dependency, uncertainty, and guilt that *we* experience in working with a person with AIDS require particular attention. Clinicians at risk for AIDS themselves face the added difficulty and responsibility of sorting through their own feelings in their work with clients. For all of us, working with very young clients who have an illness for which there is no cure, and with whom we may strongly identify, is a great challenge—and a rewarding one.

Clinicians face additional challenges. First, clients' justifiable anger at this disease—and its special psychosocial conditions—is often directed at professionals involved in their care. Clinicians need to be able to contain the anger, allow for its ventilation, and help redirect it into meaningful action when possible. Yet if a client's anger becomes abusive or disruptive, appropriate limit setting and consistent interventions must be made.

Second, since AIDS is a sexually transmitted disease, clinicians must learn to feel comfortable addressing sexuality, sexual orientation, and safe sex with clients. Most clinicians have not been trained to discuss specific behaviors with clients. If it remains too uncomfortable, clinicians must have appropriate referrals for clients to obtain the most updated information.

Fear of contagion commonly arises in every work setting in which services are provided to persons with AIDS. This fear is natural, but at times irrational. Opportunity to discuss these fears openly and obtain updated information on AIDS should help staff groups take standard infection control precautions while allaying any irrational fear. It is our responsibility as clinicians to examine our attitudes toward people in high-risk groups, in order to combat our own homophobia and fear of AIDS.

Finally, I have noticed two interesting phenomena for professionals resulting from the AIDS epidemic. First, organizations affected by AIDS can mirror death and dying themes through individual staff responses as well as organizationally. Second, because AIDS is so very new, there exists room not only for professional growth but for professional and organizational competition as well. It is incumbent upon us as professionals to monitor both these phenomena, assessing if and how they affect our effectiveness with clients.

Dan Turner: In the last five years I've witnessed many people—friends, acquaintances—facing their death. People have taken different routes. A friend of mine, a very independent man, wanted someone to be with him, and he called me. I said, fine, I'd go the next day. Well, of course, he died that night. I wasn't able to be with him. Another friend of mine committed suicide. His brother had developed AIDS and he had witnessed his brother's death, and when he was diagnosed he decided he did not want to go through that, and he elected to kill himself. People that I knew through the years—I've lived in San Francisco since the early 1970s, and of course many people I recognize on the bus or on the sidewalk—when I don't see their faces any more, I wonder what happened to them.

When I went to the clinic, I never knew whom I would run into, who would be a new person with AIDS: people from other cities who came to San Francisco for treatment because their doctors had said, "We don't have anything to give you; let's wait." By the time they got to San Francisco they were covered with lesions and they didn't really have a fighting chance. Seeing people like that really got me down.

My friend Bobbi Campbell, who, from the very beginning, wore a "Survive" button, was very courageous before he died in 1984. It wasn't until he died that I could cry, that I allowed myself to cry. I cried for myself, I cried for him. It was the first time that I really opened up and let the tears flow. Shortly after I'd been diagnosed I met Bobbi, wearing his "Survive" button. He was so courageous that it would have been wrong if I had cried. I didn't feel that I could. It wasn't until he died that I allowed myself to do so.

A friend, Paul, died this year, a very proud man, very funny. Toward the end, as his body deteriorated from KS, it was difficult for him to walk and move. I knew he had a lot of anger, but his mother came out to take care of him. To witness the two of them together, both angry and both proud—they were going to be together and make it to the end—it was wonderful to see. This woman's husband was very homophobic and did not want her to leave Texas. She was very strong. She was packing her bag and he was taking clothes out as she put them in. She grabbed a handgun and said, "Texas women have their own money, and I'm going to San Francisco to take care of my son." She did, and mother and son were really a wonderful example to everyone who witnessed them.

AIDS work for me has been therapeutic. It helped me to objectify my illness; it helped me to externalize my disease so that it would not implode in my system. I felt that the reprieve I had been given was also a responsibility, a call to arms. It was important for me to be involved, not only to stay informed but to warn my fellow gay brothers, and now the general public.

People with AIDS have been in the forefront of AIDS politics. We have been forced by an initial apathetic response to fight for our lives. Homosexuality and the diseases therein were of no consequence to the general public. They did not care for us, and so they did not care for us.

Now, after many deaths, and a threat to the nation's blood supply and military forces, they are at last willing to care.

But I wonder if there will ever be a care for *us*. We homosexuals have had to fight our own battle and care for our own. It has not been easy watching fellow fighters die, and sometimes the salutes and farewells become overwhelming. But at this point it is too late to return to a safe obscurity. One can take only mini-vacations from the ongoing tasks at hand.

After receiving calls at home from people who were newly diagnosed with AIDS, I helped to establish the People With Aids switch-board at the AIDS Foundation, so that those with AIDS would have a conduit to confer and share experiences formally with others with AIDS. The switchboard operates three hours a day, five days a week, and is manned by volunteers with AIDS. Some of those volunteers have died. A staff needs to be constantly recruited as people wear out and get sick. But the operation continues and the support of people with AIDS for people with AIDS goes on.

I have to pull away at times and take a back seat because there is only so much energy. To live with AIDS one must have the ability to say no. And to allow oneself to rest. In my MSW program at San Francisco State, for example, I decided to try other kinds of social work for my fieldwork to give myself a break from AIDS, so that I will continue to have the strength to fight it and come back at a later date, refreshed.

13

Therapy for Life, Therapy for Death

DONALD SANDNER

Sometimes in contemporary publications therapy that is directed to dying as well as staying alive is described as a recent discovery. Actually, it is an old and familiar part of the lives of tradition-oriented tribal peoples. To them birth, life, illness, and death are all bound to one meaningful whole. The Navaho, for instance, in whom I have been particularly interested, have long healing ceremonies using chants, prayers, and symbolic sand paintings. The goal of these ceremonies, properly stated, is to bring the patient into harmony with his family, his community, and his natural world. It is always hoped that the ceremony will mean restoration to a full and active life. If it does not, death is also accepted as part of the natural life of man, and though there is fear and avoidance of death, there is also respect for and recognition of it.

Those of us who do analytic work in the tradition of C. G. Jung concern ourselves with the subjective aspects of all crucial life events, including illness and death. All life events have an inner meaning, not a rational, intellectual one, but a deep, natural emotional and symbolic one, expressed by the individual psyche in spontaneous inner image and dreams. This meaning I speak of is not a collective one, but one that belongs to and can be experienced only by the individual.

It seems often that the collective rational principles of modern medicine are not enough. Scientific fact can never "prove" human values. Scientific medicine may restore the specific organ or function—and we are grateful for that—but it does not satisfy the individual, "living or dying," in his quest for balance with his surroundings and peace of mind within. As Ivan Illich says in his book *Medical Nemesis* (1976)—perhaps a bit too ungratefully: "The medical enterprise, especially when it has no clear effective remedy, sometimes saps the will of people to suffer their own reality. It destroys our ability to cope with our own bodies."

It sometimes seems that the greater enterprise of science itself portrays life as a conflict in which conquering recalcitrant nature is the only worthwhile goal. Disease and death are to be unequivocably eliminated. They can signify only defeat in the competition for unrestricted mastery of life.

But the deeper subjective psyche—the part tapped by dreams and spontaneous imagery—seems to have a different perspective. Life from beginning to end is part of an organic whole, and death is part of that wholeness. It is simply part of our "Being" in the Heideggerian sense, or of our greater "Self" in the Jungian sense, and perhaps also in the Kohutian sense. This aspect of us—our superordinate Self—is then the chief psychological factor in therapy that embraces living as completely one's Self as possible, which certainly includes death as well as birth.

In working with the inner processes I have mentioned—dreams and spontaneous inner images—it is of basic importance for the therapist to hold at bay his own preconceived opinions, his own hopes and fears, and listen with an open and receptive attitude to each individual's spontaneous productions, trusting the psyche to know its own way.

Inner healing processes come naturally into play. As Paracelsus said long ago:

> Even while still in the womb, unborn, man is burdened with the potentialities of every disease, and is subject to them. And because all diseases are inherent in his nature, he could not be born alive and healthy if an inner physician were not hidden in him. (P. 150)

Selma Hyman, professor of radiation therapy at the University of Oregon School of Medicine and a Jungian analyst, put it even more precisely in a paper about a cancer patient (1977):

> I am fully committed to scientific measures, but it is not inconsistent to believe that other dimensions to healing can be found within the individual. Medical literature contains well-documented reports of spontaneous regression of cancer and of unexpected long survivals. . . . It is my intention in my therapy to provide an atmosphere of hope with a contemporary scientific basis, and at the same time to explore archetypal measures. (P. 28)

Hyman presents a series of dreams of a forty-five-year-old woman suffering from metastatic lung carcinoma. The dreams demonstrate the inner psyche at work. There were forty dreams in all, but I would like to quote only three of them to give you the impression of the process.

Near the beginning of the analytic work came this dream:

> I am pregnant and wearing a colorfully flowered maternity bathing suit. I take off the shirt to sunbathe, and I see a big purple radiation scar on my back. I decide not to be too concerned about it. Three kittens appear and they too are pregnant. We know this by the lumps on their backs. We spend some time admiring how pretty they are and how silky, and sort of stacking them one on the other, arranging and rearranging them. (P.34)

In regard to the lumps on the kittens' back, it is noteworthy that shortly afterward metastasis in the form of lumps appeared on her lumbar vertebrae and spine; these were not visible at the time of the dream. Referring to the pregnancy of the dreamer and the kittens, Dr. Hyman says: "Psyche evidently can experience threatened death as regeneration, a phenomenon also seen in other cases. Death and renewal are closely linked symbolically" (p. 35).

> There was a large public rally where the wires for the public address system have grown and become part of a tree, like vines growing out of a heavily gnarled trunk. In the tree a metal box like a battery is found. It contains caustic rust-colored granular material that is thrown into a carp pond we are digging. I am concerned that my dog who likes to drink from the pond will be poisoned. The water is muddy but I know it will clear when the construction is done and the dust settles out. (P.35)

Here the wires and decaying metal box, which may refer to her disease (there is some resemblance to the bronchi and voicebox), are "growing into" or becoming an old gnarled tree. Also, she is preparing a pond for carp. Both the old gnarled tree and the carp are symbols of longevity or immortality. The dog, however, which she associates with her body, is threatened by the decaying metal and may be poisoned. Here we can observe how the unconscious psyche compensates and offers alternative ways of perceiving our destiny, as in the final words: "The water is muddy but I know it will clear when the construction is done."

During the months she was in therapy, much of which was agonizing and stormy, many of the long-term painful obstacles between herself and her husband cleared up. She said about her marriage: "I feel good, really good," but added wryly, "at what a price."

The last dream she recounted was that she was at the edge of a river with people standing in sneakers (but she gave them shoes that could keep them afloat in the water). She was directing a ceremony in which they held hands in a serpentine chain; interspersed in the chain were candles and food. The chain would sometimes break and she woke up crying. She could not understand why it distressed her that they wanted to be individuals apart from the interlocked chain. "This was the final preparation for entering the eternal stream. She knew it would go on, and that there would be a continuous stream even though it might sometimes break" (p. 34).

My last example is of a twenty-three-year-old young man who had developed lymphocytic lymphosarcoma when he was eighteen. His therapy included splenectomy, radiation therapy, and chemotherapy. Although there were remissions, the disease was steadily progressive.

Some time before consulting me he had a dream in which he was walking through a winding, subterranean passageway guided by a man holding a lantern. The man was an archaeologist. He guided the way to the end of the passage. There he held up the light and illuminated a partially covered Babylonian wall relief of a bearded man with wings. The bearded man reminded the dreamer of pictures he had seen of Gilgamesh, an early Sumerian mythic hero whose friendship with the untamed barbarian Enkidu was the most important emotional experience of his life. In the dream, the man with the lantern—who might represent a therapist—had quieted his fears and was now leading him underground toward the image of a deeply undeveloped masculine side of himself. The image had wings and, like its Babylonian counterpart, was connected to the spiritual.

During the last year of his life, he left college and his protected home environment to seek his independence, even though he was quite aware of the nature of his illness. He got a job in a computer industry and began to make independent emotional relationships, which he felt he had never been able to do before. At that time, he came to see me and related another dream that brought him much closer to his undeveloped darker side.

> I am in a grassy field. It's dark. Twenty young people are forming a circle in college—sort of a round dance. Suddenly there is frenzy. A big dark man pursues me and knocks me down. Then he stands over me with a long, pointed knife. He says something to me, then lets me up. I run up the grandstand as if we were in an athletic field at college. At the top was a fence and outside the stadium I see an athletic ritual of some kind. It seems to me some kind of male initiation.

The meaning of this dream—even without the association—seems remarkably clear. In the first part, he wants to join in the group of young people his own age who form a circle. But he feels left out. He still needs more intimate contact with his instinctual shadow on the inside—the dark man. In the dream, that part is real and very close to him but still threatening. Nevertheless, it contains strength and vitality. Not long after, probably impelled by his lack of time, he did unite with this inner figure.

> I am lying in my bed. There is a shadow of a man over me—forceful—full of energy—dark. He descends over me and I feel the energy come from him. It seems as if he might rape me, but then he melts into me instead. He becomes me.

Here the vitality of the dark man entered into him and filled him with the strength and courage he needed to deal with the remainder of his life.

Then his illness worsened and he had to return home. He awoke one morning shortly afterward in an intense emotional state to record a conceptual vision that he called "Death of a Programmer—The Flight of the Alone to the Alone" (Hyman 1983). In it he spoke of the "poignant contests, laughable absurdist situations" that were part of his illness, as well as the "bitterness, alienation; suppression, remission" and "inchoate liberation." Finally he wrote:

No regrets
Relaxation
Impatience, continuation
Insomnia, joy
Mechanism. Spirit tearing asunder
Making whole.
A center in the maelstrom.

As Hyman, who was seeing him at the time, said (1983, 226): "This is no picture of eternity, no vision of Elysian fields, but it is a vision of personal relation to a cosmos: a center in the maelstrom, a position earned by struggle, a sense of identity and, I believe, *meaning*."

These cases indicate that there is more to the process of dying than the outward stages charted by Kubler-Ross. There is a deeper inner process. If there is still a piece of unlived life meant to be lived, then the psyche can intensify and amplify that life so that it can be lived out in some manner—perhaps only symbolically—in the time remaining. Both of these cases show that. The woman struggled to overcome the problems in her marriage and the emotional relations with her family. The young man wanted to become strong and independent—his own man—before he died. They both succeeded.

Also, the final stage is not only acceptance. The dreams and visions here signal the connection with a deeper psychic layer, as in the woman's chain of people leading to the ocean and the young man's "center in the maelstrom." This connection brings at times a state of peace and joy, not only pain and loss. Both patients experienced this also.

In 1944, Jung had a very serious cardiac infarction and was in a deep coma, very close to death for a long time. Eventually he recovered, and I would like to close with a short excerpt from letters he wrote shortly after his recovery. Speaking of his state of near-death, he said, "In reality we know little or nothing about that mode of being, and what shall we know of this earth after death? The dissolution of our time-bound form in eternity brings no loss of meaning. Rather does the little finger then know itself a member of the hand" (Adler 1984, 53) and "Death is the hardest thing from the outside and as long as we are outside of it. But once inside you taste of such completeness and peace and fulfillment that you don't want to return" (p. 60).

References

Hyman, S. 1977. *Death in life, life in death—Spontaneous process in a cancer patient*. New York: Spring Publications.

———. 1983. Therapeutic use of spontaneous imagery. *Perspectives in Bio and Med* 26 (2):226.

Illich, I. 1976. *Medical nemesis*. New York: Random House.

Jung, C. G. 1984. *Selected letters of C. G. Jung, 1909–1961*, ed. Gerhard Adler. Princeton: Bollingen Series, Princeton University Press.

Paracelsus. 1951. *Selected writings*. New York: Pantheon.

PART III

Related Issues

14

Reflections on Archetypal Aspects of AIDS and a Psychology of Gay Men

SCOTT WIRTH

I dedicate my comments to my dear friend, Lyle Dobson, who died of AIDS in April 1985, and to the eight other mental health professionals known to me who have died of AIDS or are suffering from it.

One of the worst feelings many of us have had about AIDS stems from our sense of its arbitrariness, its impenetrability, its cruelty, and its medical unyieldingness—no treatment, no medical cure, no end in sight to the epidemic. In a sense, the medical intransigence of AIDS leaves us no choice but to work with the psyche—over that, at least, it seems we have some measure of influence. Whether our focus is to prevent the development of new AIDS cases or to counsel those who already have AIDS, our immediate hopes rest largely on changing consciousness about the disease, rather than eliminating the disease itself.

Let us take as an example the familiar, urgent, and behaviorally concrete task of changing mass-scale awareness of gay male sexual practices, in other words the internalization and integration of safe sex guidelines throughout the gay men's community. For all the impressive educational campaigns and massive turnarounds in sexual behavior that we have seen in only a few years' time, a significant number of gay men destructively continue to put themselves and one another at life risk. The AIDS virus is being dispersed into our collective pool of bodily fluids faster than our expeditious educational efforts can prevent it.

Most gay men in San Francisco now know the informational do's and don'ts of safe sex conduct. Although I wholeheartedly support all mass advertising-style educational campaigns, I believe that the education/advertising model is insufficient by itself. A gay man's survival from now into the foreseeable future will have more to do with his psychological capacity to extract and personally internalize the information he already has than it will with having new and improved information in his fund of knowledge. Each gay man needs to approach AIDS prevention individually and in psychological depth. His ability not just to survive but to individuate and thrive will depend on his looking deeply within himself, including into the meanings of his sexual history and sexual identity.

AIDS has precipitated a crisis in community that is unspeakably traumatic yet presents untold opportunities for both self-knowledge and knowledge of intimate relationship. Such discovery is a highly individualized matter. I have, nevertheless, found it fruitful for myself as a psychologist to consider some broad themes of the psychology of gay men. I would like to share some of my reflections in the spirit of open inquiry rather than as fixed assumptions or established truths. My scope will be limited to men—not to exclude the importance of directly comparing a psychology of gay men with that of women, but simply because of space constraints.

I will be using some of the language of analytical psychology and in particular the term "archetype." For those unfamiliar with this term I offer an explanatory passage from Jean Shinoda Bolen's book, *Goddesses in Everywoman* (1984):

> C. G. Jung introduced the concept of archetypes into psychology. He saw archetypes as patterns of instinctual behavior that were contained in a collective unconscious. The collective unconscious is the part of the unconscious that is not individual but universal, with contents and modes of behavior that are more or less the same everywhere and in all individuals.
>
> Myths and fairy tales are expressions of archetypes, as are many images and themes in dreams. The presence of common archetypal patterns in all people accounts for similarities in the mythologies of many different cultures. As preexistent patterns, they influence how we behave and how we react to others. (P. 15)

In many ways, gay men share common ground with other men. I believe, however, that gay men are also different, both graced and vexed with an early and fuller access to two realms of male consciousness. One realm, quite obviously, is the homoerotic, which in Jungian archetypal terms might be personified in the form of the Greek god Pan. The second realm is the inner Feminine, in Jungian archetypal terms the anima. I would like to conjecture that for most gay men the encounter with these two archetypal dimensions constitutes a central task of individuation, or psychological development. Further, when an unconscious relationship to the homoerotic or to the Feminine exists within a given gay male, the psychic energies of these extraordinarily potent archetypal influences can lead to a destructive life course, a "takeover," so to speak, by what Jung called the "mana personality." In the section of his essay "The Relations Between the Ego and the Unconscious" (1935), which deals with the mana personality, Jung writes:

> It is indeed hard to see how one can escape the sovereign power of the primordial images. Actually, I do not believe it can be escaped. One can only alter one's attitude and thus save oneself from naively falling into an archetype and being forced to act a part at the expense of one's humanity. Possession by an archetype turns a man into a flat collective figure, a mask behind which he can no longer develop as a human being. (P.234)

I would add that—at least in the case of some gay men—possession by an archetype can also create such an unconscious relationship to one's own sexuality and identity that the person is caught in compulsive patterns and self-destructive currents that can endanger health and even life itself. Regrettably, I cannot here reflect on gay men's relationship to the inner Feminine, the anima; rather, I will concentrate on discussing the homoerotic.

Let us conjecture that homosexuality is indeed an archetypal expression of the human organism. Its libidinal presence may be strong or weak; it may be lived out, consciously sublimated, or only imagined in thought or fantasy. We see images of the homoerotic in all times and places, everywhere from ancient Greek mythology to the sports pages of our daily newspapers.

Without probing into reasons why, let us acknowledge that gay men *express* the human capacity for loving sensuality between males. Actually, in modern times and in major urban centers such as San Francisco, gay male sensuality is characteristically full, lively, and open. Drawing from the imagery of Greek mythology, we might say that in the openly sexual lives of modern gay men we recognize an affinity with Pan, the wild god of woods and fields.

Pan amused himself with the chase; he led the dances of the nymphs. Close to communal animal life—to flocks, herds, and beehives—he boasted that he had coupled orgiastically with each of Dionysus's drunken Maenads. According to Kerenyi, he is the great phallic god who, "when he originally came into being, had only a single twin brother and represented the darker half of a divine male couple" (1979, 174). Hermes carried Pan up to Olympus for the gods' amusement, though he was not included as one of the Olympian twelve. He was creative, the inventor of the syrinx, or shepherd's pipe, which he played in a masterly manner. And, very significantly, he was the only god to die in our time.

To return to our mortal psychology, we can intuitively recognize aspects of today's gay man in Pan. Let us consider not only the possibility that some gay men are hazardously possessed by the Pan archetype but that this psychological imbalance is further complicated by the collective psychosocial problems of men in modern society. In other words, in the San Francisco of the mid-1980s we are not cavorting through the woods dancing with nymphs. Quite the contrary.

The frank and even exuberant expression of homoeroticism among gay males calls forth varying degrees of inner, unconscious envy, anxiety, fear, and aggression among many nongay males. These nongay men may manage their inner conflict by employing such familiar mechanisms of defense as projection and denial to distance themselves from their own homoerotic impulses, fantasies, or feelings. The majority of males split off the homosexual component of their own human potential, attributing it to a distinct group of "homosexuals," who then also are scapegoated* and even wantonly denigrated.

Thus we find that homosexual the adjective, the human quality, becomes homosexual the noun, the group, the other-than-myself. Gay men become the sexual shadow of nongay men, appearing to them in their unconscious fantasies of gay men as the Satyr, the Devil, Pan, Dionysus, the Fool, the Queen. Gay men are unconsciously regarded as dangerously handsome, potent, pleasure-laden, and lustful. Gay men are consciously considered inferior sexual beings—deviant, animalistic, childlike, sick, sinful, and womanly.

Certainly everyone can think of examples from everyday life that illustrate the psychological dynamics of scapegoating that I'm describing. If it were only so easy to say simply that the unaware, repressed nongay patriarchs are oppressing the innocent, joyful gay brother-

---

*The word *scapegoat* is curious in reference to Pan, for he possessed the horns, beard, tail, and legs of a goat.

hood! This naive, even at times adolescent, unconscious identification with the role of innocent and persecuted victim has led some gay men to neglect the difficult work of consciously integrating the psyche. In his role of oppressed victim, a gay man may keep himself immature until the straight patriarch comes around. The bad father has failed. Where, asks the naive gay man, is the good father who will superintend this awful earthly place so unfriendly to youthful gayety?

Possessed and identified with the archetype of eternal youth, the *puer aeternus*, he reacts unaware against the negative father. He becomes a sexual figurine. He mirrors the rejecting father's splitting off and denial of the homoerotic by isolating sex in his own genitals, separating instinct from thought, divorcing sexual experience from the emotional, relational aspects of life.

Seeking approval, gratification, excitement, a short cut to self-esteem, he flies high (on drugs or otherwise) only to collapse and fall like Icarus. Or, looking for perfect love, he misses the opportunity for actual relationship, caught in a circle of fantasies, gazing like Narcissus into his own eyes.

Sitting with gay patients for many years since the birth of the gay liberation movement, I sensed collective developmental patterns of change even before AIDS proliferated in our community. I felt from patients a sense of emptiness and boredom with the sexual sport. I heard an acknowledgment, with a chuckle or a weary sigh, that many gay men had experienced just about every sexual activity in every environmental scenario with every mind-altering substance that existed. We had finally had that ten-year adolescence that we had missed in the first place. *All* of it: peer pressure, wardrobe, fads, cliques, hangouts, competition, body awkward/body beautiful, testing of limits, cult figures and heroes, rebellion, god, idealism, *all* of it. Even, at last, the gym!

AIDS, we might say, is the end of paradise. The bubble has popped. It is a shock, it is horrible, depressing, and disillusioning. But deep down inside no one is completely surprised. And in some sense we feel relieved. It is time to change, to move on to a new stage. We can never forget our adolescence, nor do we wish to forget it. Whether we actively participated or only observed this time of our lives, we hope to carry threads from this period into the future. Already, there is nostalgia for the "good old days" before AIDS. This child, this youth is precious—he is inside us now forever.

But there is also a reluctance to go on. Another Pan, *Peter* Pan, does not want to grow up. Ah! The freedom, the gratification, the highs, the drama, the excitement of rapid growth! A narcissistic sense of unfairness wells up, a last rebellious touch, a clinging to the charm of it all.

Our natural, chronological adolescence was arrested by culture and society. Our fully experienced youth was delayed by circumstances beyond our control. As we grieve the loss of our loved ones to AIDS, simultaneously we grieve the loss of an era: the birth, growth, and coming of age of our gay selves. In some odd way, AIDS helps us to grow. Crazily—and the root word "crazy" derives from the old Norwegian *krasa*, which means crushed or fragmented—crazily, AIDS first crushes us, then invites and impels us to reintegrate, to make ourselves whole again in a new way. This thing called AIDS, this virus, these microbes are the face of another archetype, the Great Mother, who is at once good and bad, who makes possible a union of negative and positive, who devours and creates. Antonin Artaud, whom some regarded as crazy, wrote a poem in 1947 after the A-bombs and death camps of his time. Titled "To Have Done With The Judgement of God" (1975), it reads:

> for, laugh as much as you want to,
> what men have called microbes is in fact god,
> and do you know what the Americans and the Russians
> make their bombs with?
> They make them with the microbes of god.

Anyone who comes close to AIDS can be emotionally overcome, inundated or inflated by the mystery and power of the pain beyond words, flooded with the enormity of it all, the ego overwhelmed by the contents of the collective unconscious. From an archetypal psychological viewpoint the god Pan may present himself again. About this aspect of him we read in Bulfinch (1978, 166) that

> Pan, like other gods who dwelt in forests, was dreaded by those whose occupations caused them to pass through the woods by night, for the gloom and loneliness of such scenes dispose the mind to superstitious fears. Hence sudden fright without any visible cause was ascribed to Pan and called a Panic terror.

It is easy to identify the panic about AIDS of nurses at San Francisco General Hospital or parents in Queens, New York. *

---

*Near the time of the conference presentation, September 1985, newspapers carried accounts of a group of nurses at San Francisco General Hospital who were reprimanded by

It is harder to be aware of the bargaining we health professionals engage in with our own feelings of powerlessness and unconscious panic at those moments of countertransference when in working with AIDS patients we are inflated by the mana personality, experiencing ourselves as the doctor hero, the priestly counselor, or the overnight psychic.

It is by becoming conscious of the hitherto unconscious contents of the psyche that one becomes what Jung (1935) called "psychologically housetrained." He wrote that

> the dissolution of the mana personality comes about through the conscious assimilation of its contents, which leads us, by a natural route, back to ourselves as an actual living something, poised between two world pictures and their darkly discerned potencies. This "something" is strange to us and yet so near, wholly ourselves and yet unknowable. (P. 237)

Reading this passage, I thought of one theme of this volume—Helping people live, helping people die. Perhaps these are the two world pictures between which we as mental health practitioners are poised.

Part of why it is such a privilege to know and to work with people dying from AIDS is that often they are such practical exemplars of the process of freeing oneself from unconscious attachments, of meeting change step by step. Jung stressed that the natural way to approach death is to live life fully, to continue to live as if life continued forever. Donald Sandner in his book *Navajo Symbols of Healing* (1979) writes that

> one idea running through all mythological systems is that life goes on forever and is constantly subjected to renewal; death is only a regrettable interlude. . . . Such beliefs are not, or need not be, directly connected with ideas of an afterlife that involves reward or punishment. They are merely the deep-seated archetypal belief in the continuation of life. (P. 255)

It is my observation that men with AIDS realize this quite directly. Many gay men have their own children or have nieces or nephews to

---

hospital officials and then sued the hospital for their refusal to work with AIDS patients without using protective masks, gowns, and gloves whenever they chose. Also, in Queens, N.Y., parents and children staged demonstrations and organized a boycott of public elementary schools calling for the quarantine of children with AIDS from classrooms. Yet expert medical opinion consistently maintains that AIDS cannot be spread through casual contact.

whose futures they look as a connection to the ongoing stream of life.
Most men with AIDS, however, find their relationship to the archetype of continuation in other ways. It may simply mean staying at
home, not in a hospital, carrying on the rounds of domestic life as well
as possible, perhaps becoming closer to friends. It may mean recon-
ciliation with estranged family members; pursuing alternative methods
of self-healing; participating in research experiments either to benefit
one's own recovery or to contribute to a possible scientific break-
through that will benefit others. AIDS may provide a spiritual opening
to meditation or prayer. It can open a path of political activism, lobbying for AIDS funds or doing volunteer work with persons with AIDS.

Someone in the terminal stages of AIDS may choose to make a personal statement by consciously and intentionally taking control of his
own dying process, choosing the time and circumstance of his own
death—and perhaps in so doing affecting medical and legal opinion
about the right to die without pain and with dignity. Allowing others
to care for him may permit another man finally to feel himself loved
and accepted as never before. Some gay men may use their AIDS diagnosis as an opportunity for coming out to others, thus advancing
awareness of homosexuality in society.

Through all these expressions runs the archetypal belief in the continuation of life. We also see in many of these life examples the devastation of AIDS rendered personally meaningful. This makes all the
difference, for as Sandner writes in the opening chapter of *Navajo
Symbols of Healing*: "Man can accept a tremendous amount of legiti-
mate suffering; what he cannot accept is suffering that has no purpose.
To be endured and accepted, suffering must be given a meaning"
(p. 11).

References

Artaud, A. 1975. To have done with the judgement of God. Trans. Clayton
    Eshleman and Norman Glass. *Sparrow #34*. Los Angeles: Black Sparrow
    Press.

Bolen, J. S. 1984. *Goddesses in everywoman: A new psychology of women*. San
    Francisco: Harper & Row.

Bulfinch, T. 1978. The rural deities. In *Bulfinch's mythology*. New York: Avenel
    Books.

Jung, C. G. 1935. The relations between the ego and the unconscious. 2d ed. In *Collected Works of C. G. Jung*. Vol. 7. Princeton: Princeton University Press, 1966.

Kerenyi, C. 1979. The birth and love-affairs of Pan. In *The gods of the Greeks*, trans. Norman Cameron. New York: Thames & Hudson.

Sandner, D. 1979. *Navajo symbols of healing*. New York: Harcourt Brace Jovanovich.

15

Women and AIDS

NANCY SHAW AND LYN PALEO

In 1983 the first brochure on women and AIDS was produced. Since then a great deal has happened. With the growing awareness that women can contract AIDS has come the realization of needs: that specialized services should be provided to them and that health care providers will increasingly come into contact with women who have some kind of AIDS concern. Some women may have been exposed to AIDS, others have close friends or family members who are ill. Additionally, many of the health care personnel providing AIDS services are women.

Women At Risk: Epidemiology

AIDS in women presents a different epidemiological pattern from that found among men. The most prevalent risk category is IV drug use (53 percent), according to CDC AIDS activity reports. The next category, or group of women with AIDS, is one for which no root of transmission has been identified, referred to as "none/other" by the CDC (20 percent) (1986). Included in this risk category are women from countries where a higher proportion of the population has AIDS or ARC or may be seropositive. This includes women diagnosed in the United States who immigrated here from Haiti and Zaire. For many of the women (including the nonimmigrants) in the "none/other" category, the probable risk factor was heterosexual contact with a man who was infected with the virus but is not in an identified risk group. His infection may have been through a person that he did not know to be in a risk category (for example, his wife, who had a blood transfusion prior to his meeting her).

Another grouping of women in the "none/other" category is composed of those who were diagnosed late in their illness or only at autopsy. Because men and their health care providers are more aware of the possibility of contracting AIDS, male diagnoses may take place at earlier stages. This allows more time for adequate investigation into the source of infection. If more women are diagnosed only at autopsy, risk factors will be more difficult to determine. Systematic research has not yet been conducted into this issue. It is striking, however, that in only a very small percentage of male AIDS cases is "none/other" listed for patient groups.

Another aspect of surveillance that may affect the female "none/other" category is that the questions listed on the CDC surveillance form are not designed to elicit special data on female risk groups. Data are collected on "homosexuality," for example, but the word "lesbian" is not used. Many health care providers are not aware that their female patients may be lesbians. Consequently, this risk factor may be overlooked. In a similar vein, questions are not asked about donor insemination, although clinical reports demonstrate clearly the possibility of viral transmission via insemination.

The third risk category is heterosexual contact. Even though many more men than women have AIDS, for about five times as many women as men is heterosexual contact the suspected route of infection, according to the CDC. One reason for this difference is that, regardless of initial route of infection (for example, gay activity, hemophilia, drug use, transfusion), there are more males currently carrying the virus than females. This means that in terms of heterosexual contact, more males are capable of transmitting the virus.

A second consideration may be that AIDS is more readily transmissible from males to females than vice versa. Additionally, some heterosexual contact includes anal intercourse, an important risk factor for virus transmission. Research in *types* of heterosexual activity and virus transmission has yet to be completed. Within the heterosexual risk category, the partners of the women were predominantly IV drug users (72 percent); bisexual men as partners are a much smaller group (19 percent) (Hardy 1985).

The fourth risk category for women is transfusions with blood or blood products, according to the CDC. It accounts for 9 percent of all female cases. New cases from earlier transfusions will continue to appear, but the risk of transfusion-related transmission is currently near zero.

A fifth risk category for women is "hemophiliac/coagulation disorder." Four adult females were in this category in 1986. Women *do* have coagulation disorders for which they receive the same types of blood products as are prescribed for hemophiliacs. As with transfusions, the current risk associated with Factor VII blood products is essentially zero.

In California, women's risk factors are somewhat different from the national ones. Transfusion-related AIDS is a more common cause of infection than drug use. Drug use and heterosexual contact are the second most important risk factors (California Health Services 1986). Of the California women who contracted AIDS through heterosexual contact, two of them had partners who were both IV drug users *and* bisexual. One had a partner who was an IV drug user, one had a partner who was homosexual/bisexual, one partner was a hemophiliac, and about two we do not have adequate data. In California, as of September 1985, two lesbians were identified with AIDS diagnoses. One contracted it through a transfusion, the other via IV drug use (Miller 1985).

These data refer to AIDS cases only. We estimate that there are ten times as many ARC cases and one hundred times as many women who are infected.

In California, female AIDS cases are concentrated in several of the larger metropolitan areas: Los Angeles, San Francisco, and Alameda County, for example. Although surveillance figures are *supposed* to refer to the county of *residence*, they actually represent the county of *diagnosis*. In some cases, but not all, the county of residence is the same. This fact should be taken into account when services are being developed and when city and county budgets are being prepared.

There is no evidence that prostitutes constitute a special risk category. The CDC documented this, as has preliminary research being done in San Francisco (Wofsy et al. 1986, Schultz et al. 1986, Wykoff 1986). Some prostitutes do get AIDS. To the extent that researchers have been able to isolate prostitution and/or multiple sexual contacts from such issues as IV drug use, however, neither the number of sexual contacts nor the receipt of money for sex (by sex therapists, prostitutes, call girls, and the like) seems to put women at a higher risk for getting AIDS. Many women who are in paid sexual activity were concerned about sexually transmitted diseases even before the AIDS epidemic. They protected themselves and continue to protect themselves by being somewhat alert to new medical developments in sexually transmitted diseases and how to avoid them. They may be better protected than the typical woman who is "just going to a bar" or a woman who thinks of herself as not sexually active but who "just happens to have this relationship." They may be more aware than women who are involved in serial monogamy or those whose self-image is "I'm not at risk so I'm not going to learn more about it."

Transmission and Its Prevention

Prevention of HIV transmission for women is essentially the same as it is for gay men and will be described below. The safe sex guidelines, now in use with gay men, can, with a little creativity, be revised to apply to women. AIDS is caused by a virus transmitted in some, but not all, bodily secretions. It can be *found* in probably every bodily secretion, including blood, spinal fluid, semen, saliva, sweat, and tears. But that does *not* mean it can be transmitted via all these routes. The concentration varies significantly from fluid to fluid. The highest concentrations are in blood, spinal fluid, and semen. Even when traces of the virus are found in other fluids, saliva, for instance, they may be in a nontransmissible or poorly transmissible form. The concentration may also be too low for effective transmission.

The virus *can* be transmitted through blood, as epidemiological data indicate, and through semen. Those are the two main bodily fluids to be wary of. Blood can appear in a variety of places. One could have blood in her saliva; in that case, then, her saliva might be an effective transmission route. Blood often passes through the colon as a matter of course, without any illness being present. It is often in feces and there may be fecal contact in sexual activity, either advertently or inadvertently. Blood is also present in menstrual fluid, which can be in smaller or larger amounts in vaginal and/or cervical secretions.

Although numerous studies about transmission of the virus during sexual activities between men are in progress, little research has been completed on sexual transmission and women (with either a heterosexual or lesbian focus). Finding HIV in vaginal secretions does not answer the question of vaginal transmission. For that we need an epidemiological study. One epidemiological study addressing this issue is the AWARE study at UCSF, under the direction of Constance Wofsy and Judith Cohen (1986). Very few of the participants thus far have positive antibody test results, indicating infection. All these women, however, were IV drug users in addition to being at risk through sexual contact. The study (ultimately of 500 women at risk) will give us extensive data concerning virus transmission.

A second epidemiological study of women and AIDS in San Francisco, conducted by Nancy Padian, focuses on the female sexual partners of gay and bisexual men (1986). The men's blood has been analyzed for seroconversion since 1980. The female partners of a sample of the men are being tested for HIV antibody positivity.

The third San Francisco epidemiological project on AIDS transmission and women is the Lesbian Insemination Project (LIP), affiliated with the AWARE study (Pies 1986). LIP's purpose is to gather more information about semen as a transmitter of the virus when the factor of sexual intercourse is removed. The subjects in this study have a very low rate of sexual activity with men, but they have been exposed to semen through donor insemination. The project investigates antibody positivity in the women and, in some cases, their children.

Research results are important to educators and health care providers who wish to provide accurate information to their clients concerning transmission and prevention of AIDS. Our approach—in this field where so little is known—is to base our education on as much knowledge as we can and to make conservative recommendations, erring on the side of safety.

For most sexual activity—vaginal intercourse, anal intercourse, and fellatio—the most important AIDS transmission risk is semen entering the body. The best prevention method is condoms. Condoms do seem to act as an effective barrier to the virus, just as they act as a barrier to almost every other virus. Condoms can be used in any kind of intercourse and in fellatio by mutual agreement or, in fact, without it. Many prostitutes and other women in the sex industry use condoms without their clients knowing it. The woman holds the condom in her mouth until she performs fellatio and, with a learned skill and ease, puts it on the man and takes it off after the act is finished. He never knows.

Transmission may also occur when sex toys are shared. Any item (dildo or vibrator, for example) should *not* be used internally by both partners. If it is, it should be cleaned with bleach, alcohol, or hydrogen peroxide.

Previous exposure and current sexual activity are two separate factors. If two people are at very "high risk" because of their previous practices, they still could be presently engaging in very safe sexual activities, including use of condoms. Conversely, they may be two people whose sexual activities have been very limited, or they may have been monogamous for years. They do not *have* a sexual risk factor, yet they are very worried: "Well, everyone's pointing the finger at us, saying we're going to get AIDS, because we engage in anal intercourse, and *they* say that's how the gay men get it."

Another aspect of risk is dose. Researchers believe that repeated doses of the virus are sometimes necessary for infection. One might have a brush with the virus, some contact with it, and not *necessarily* become infected. But infection *could* also occur after only one exposure.

An effective lubricant, gel, or spermicide to use with a condom is nonoxynol-9, which kills HIV in laboratory settings (Hicks et al.

1985). This does not necessarily guarantee that it will kill the virus in other settings. Home use is different from clinical studies. We cannot say categorically to a client, "If you use nonoxynol-9, you will be safe." It will, however, lower the risk of transmission. Nonoxynol-9 lubricants can be applied both inside and outside a condom. Some condoms are also prelubricated with spermicide. Using a condom appropriately, without user error, breakage, and so forth, *will* prevent the virus from entering the body during ejaculation (Conant et al. 1985). So, in terms of intercourse, even fellatio, the condom is a very effective protective device.

Basically, safe sex boils down to one concept: "Do not allow one person's semen, blood, feces, vaginal secretions, or, in the case of lactating mothers, mother's milk, into another person's body." That might mean using condoms; it might mean not ejaculating. Vaginal secretions may also transmit the virus. If a woman were infected, cunnilingus *might* transmit the virus to her partner.

To prevent a partner's exposure to her menstrual blood and/or cervical secretions, a woman can use a diaphragm and nonoxynol-9, and have her partner use a condom. Such activity reduces, but does not eliminate, the risk of transmission.

Another aspect of sexual transmission is saliva and kissing. Saliva poses a difficult question for the health educator and mental health care provider. It is quite easy to prove that something does transmit a virus; all you need is one case in which it has. It is much more difficult to prove that it does not. In all likelihood, saliva does *not* transmit the AIDS virus, unless there is blood mixed in with it. Brushing your teeth or having cuts or sores in your mouth can produce blood. If the virus is in the blood, it is then "in" the saliva. But saliva itself (or with minute amounts of blood) has never been implicated in a case of HIV transmission. The viral concentration is apparently too low. Some comparisons have been made between HIV and the hepatitis B virus, which is, similarly, transmitted primarily through blood and semen. Hepatitis B virus is also found in saliva, but in thirty years of research not one case has been linked to salival transmission. As health care providers, we must be alert to the client who says, "Oh well, saliva's probably risky, and so is semen, and I'm not going to stop kissing, so I might as well not stop intercourse without a condom." Semen is *known* to transmit the virus.

Levels of Risk

Communities and populations have variable rates of virus exposure. In the case of a community like the gay male community of San Francisco (with a 50 percent infection rate) or the New York IV drug user community (with as many as 80 percent of the community exposed), the basic public health goals should be that everybody engage only in safe sex, for protection of self and others. Community survival will require major behavioral changes.

In a community where the incidence of infection is below 50 percent, perhaps only 1 percent, the average person is less likely to want to use condoms. How can one mandate safe sex for *everyone*? If one follows the risk reduction guidelines in all cases, there would be no pregnancies. One aspect of sexual counseling for the lower risk population is education on decision making and risk evaluation. The client should be asked, "What level of risk are you willing to take?" Some people feel that they have very little risk of exposure and that their partner has little or no risk. They feel safe, or safe enough to do "everything." Some people review their pasts and those of their partners. Others take antibody tests and then decide about sex. Still others take the attitude that if there's any risk at all, they would rather avoid sex. Some risks are more acceptable than others to an individual. One person will drive drunk, but always use a condom. Another is the reverse. Partners negotiate to what degree each wishes to take some sort of risk.

Pregnancy and Pediatric Issues

Most pediatric AIDS patients (77 percent) contracted the illness via a parent with AIDS or at increased risk for AIDS, as of June 1986, 224 infants, 114 male and 110 female (CDC 1986). Although there is a chance of the fetus being exposed to the virus through transplacental transmission *in utero*, not every baby will be born infected (Scott et al. 1985). In some cases, infected women who have given birth to infected children have later delivered noninfected, healthy children. We cannot predict whether a specific infant will be born infected. Additionally, some children who have had positive results on the AIDS antibody tests remain in good health. Transmission of the virus can also occur via breast milk. A clinical report from Australia identified one infant who became antibody-positive after its mother received a tainted blood transfusion postnatally and then nursed her child over a period of months (Ziegler et al. 1985).

If a woman is infected at the start of a pregnancy, what are her chances of developing the symptoms of ARC or AIDS during the course of pregnancy? Pregnancy may accelerate the course of illnesses associated with AIDS and ARC and perhaps also the underlying syndrome itself. Counseling women who are already pregnant, and at the point when abortion is feasible, is a complex and difficult task (San Francisco Public Health Department 1986).

And lastly, donor insemination. No women who received semen via donor insemination have yet contracted AIDS. One study in Australia demonstrated that the virus is transmissible via insemination. Freezing the sperm may make transmission less likely. Screening programs similar to those in use in blood banks are the major technique for preventing transmission via insemination. Typically, a sexual and social history of the donor, blood tests, and other screens are used. HIV antibody tests are in routine use at licensed sperm banks.

Testing for the antibody to HIV is a screening strategy that is being increasingly applied as a protection even beyond the blood banking community. Sperm banks use it. Some doctors recommend it for their patients considering pregnancy. Some people want it to feel secure about their sexual activity. While the test is relatively accurate, it is not 100 percent perfect. Since we are dealing with a potentially deadly illness, the imperfections of the test are very important to understand.

The consequence of a false-negative result is that a woman may *wrongly* think that she is not carrying the virus and spread it inadvertently or misunderstand her real symptoms of AIDS or ARC. In most testing systems, negative test results are not a signal to retest and the result is treated as "true." Any woman in a high-risk group who gets an initial negative result should consider a retest for certainty.

The consequence of a false-positive result can be unnecessary stress, anxiety, and fear. Because almost all testing programs include retests of positive specimens, any woman with an initial positive test is likely to have her blood retested automatically. Retesting significantly reduces the risk of a false result.

Women's Unique Issues

First, there is the problem of maternal transmission, already described. Women at risk for infection are going to be counseled about pregnancy, abortion, breastfeeding, contraception, and antibody tests. They are going to be encouraged to share information about their antibody status with obstetricians, labor room staffs, and pediatricians. Some may even be told to delay pregnancy indefinitely "until more is known." How will women react to such advice?

In some cities, women in high-risk groups are being encouraged to have antibody testing prior to pregnancy. It is entirely possible that women, or subgroups of them, and not gay men, will be the first population to face mass screening for the AIDS virus antibody.

A second aspect of AIDS that is unique to women is the social role of mothering: From this role flow two important consequences. First, when a woman becomes ill with ARC or AIDS, her role as a primary care-giver to a child or children or to other adults in the household is immediately affected. The family is severely disrupted, and she herself will have to make many adjustments. Her children may also be indirectly affected by her diagnosis and forbidden to go to school. She has to deal with a life-threatening illness, and she also has to deal with the impact on her family, and this is a very serious matter. As stated earlier, 53 percent of women with AIDS contracted it through IV drug use. A significant number got it through heterosexual contact, most often with a drug user. Demographic studies of such women indicate that they are likely to have young children and also to be the sole support of these children.

A second consequence of the social role of motherhood is care of the child with AIDS. With AIDS, as with other sicknesses, it is ordinarily the mother who is expected to care for or manage the care of the child. But since most pediatric AIDS cases are the result of maternal transmission, the mother may herself be ill. Her illness and responsibility may be compounded by illegal survival activity, incarceration, poor health (caused by drug use and illnesses associated with its life-style), and the threat of foster care or child abuse proceedings. These are parenting issues that men rarely face.

If the mother is healthy enough to care for her child, she must still handle the complex issues of medical and home care, research investigations, school access, friends, and family stress. CDC recommends that every child be evaluated individually to provide quality care for a child who either is infected with the virus or is ill (Education and Foster Care 1985).

Resources for Women

Because the total number of women infected with HIV is much smaller than the number of men, the general resources available for women and those that deal with particular problems of women are much more limited. Let us look briefly at the area of drug rehabilitation services— necessary to combat AIDS transmission via shared needles. Both in absolute numbers, and in proportion to need, fewer drug programs exist for women than for men (Shaw 1985). Residential programs have fewer spaces available for women than for men. In addition, most of the programs will not take women who are pregnant, and those that will take women who are pregnant will not take them when they are more than twenty-one weeks pregnant. None will house a woman with a child.

The only residential substance abuse program in San Francisco that will take women who are pregnant and/or have children is the Women's Alcoholism Center, which requires that the woman's primary problem be alcohol, not drugs. As a consequence, a woman with a drug problem who is at risk for AIDS and has children is forced to leave her children in order to be treated in a residential program. She probably will not be able to have visitors, including her children, for at least two months. Such rules are standard in many residential programs. These programs are designed to meet men's needs, not those of women.

Women need AIDS services as well. Many AIDS-focused organizations have no women's support group or people who are particularly sensitive to women's issues. Organization members, clinic staff, and health department employees may be sensitive to the issues of AIDS in a general way, but many are not trained to understand those problems specific to women.

Another aspect of resources and services for women is the need for ethnic diversity in staff and programs. Most female AIDS cases are black or Latino women. Effective educational programs require culturally sensitive and linguistically appropriate materials, combined with active outreach. This is not happening so far any place in the United States. Work with local ethnic health and civic organizations can be an important step in raising community awareness of AIDS and preventive techniques and assist those affected. Most women with AIDS are from poor backgrounds. As a whole, they are probably poorer than men with AIDS. This means that more resources are going to be needed for women than for men.

At the 1985 International Conference on AIDS in Atlanta, many researchers discussing sexuality would refer to sexually active men and promiscuous women. Prostitutes were described as "a reservoir of infections" (Schultz et al. 1986, Wykoff 1986, Redfield et al. 1986). Just as gay men are stigmatized for their sexual activity, so women who cannot prove that they contracted the virus from their husbands or from blood transfusions are also going to be stigmatized and criticized and blamed for their (imagined) sex life and morals.

Women as Health Care Providers

Numerically, women constitute the bulk of the care-giving population for those who have AIDS. Persons with AIDS are primarily men. The medical care system itself is dominated by men. This situation mirrors women's family role of filling others' physical and emotional needs and being responsible for their daily maintenance. Many of us are in the situation of providing extensive service but receiving inadequate recognition. We have the role (which we have filled for centuries) of caring for the sick, handling emotional problems, handling issues of nurturance, doing the daily work, doing the dirty work, handling everybody's waste materials in one form or another, being exposed. The AIDS epidemic makes our nurturing roles more necessary while simultaneously reducing our self-worth. If we begin to complain about, for example, sexism or lack of recognition, we are told, or may tell ourselves, that we are dealing with a very serious epidemic, we're talking about people dying, and after all, I am a woman who is not at much risk. "I'm healthy, what right have I to ask for anything?"

We experience this criticism externally and internally. On the one hand, women have frustrations about status in the hierarchical structures of medicine; and on the other hand, they feel that they should not complain. Therefore, meeting the challenges of the AIDS epidemic may include addressing the role of women health care professionals as well as the needs of women at risk of illness.

References

California Department of Health Services, Office of AIDS. 1986. *Acquired immunodeficiency syndrome monthly field activities report.* April 30.

Centers for Disease Control. 1986. *Acquired immunodeficiency syndrome weekly surveillance report.* June 2.

Conant, M., D. Hardy, J. Sernatinger, et al. 1986. Condoms prevent transmission of AIDS-associated retrovirus. *JAMA* 255:1706.

Education and foster care of children infected with human T-lymphotropic virus type III/lymphadenopathy-associated virus. 1985. *MMWR* 34:517–21.

Hardy, A. 1985. Centers for Disease Control, personal communication, September 9.

Hicks, D. R., L. S. Martin, J. P. Getchell, et al. 1985. Inactivation of HTLV-III/LAV-infected cultures of normal human lymphocytes by nonoxynol-9 in vitro. *Lancet* 2:1422.

Miller, D. 1985. California Department of Health Services, personal communication, September 9.

Padian, N. 1986. Preliminary data presented at APHA meeting, November. Washington, D.C.

Pies, C. 1986. Preliminary data presented at International Conference on AIDS, June 23–25. Paris, France.

Redfield, R. R., D. C. Wright, P. D. Markham, et al. 1986. Letter to the editor. *JAMA* 255:1705–6.

San Francisco Department of Public Health, Perinatal and Pediatric AIDS Advisory Committee. 1986. Guidelines for control of perinatally transmitted human T-lymphotropic virus-type III/lymphadenopathy-associated virus infection and care of infected mothers, infants and children. *SF Epid Bull* 2, supplement 1, April.

Schultz, S., J. A. Milberg, A. R. Kristal, R. L. Stoneburner. 1986. Female to male transmission of HTLV-III. *JAMA* 255:1703–4.

Scott, G. B., M. A. Fischl, N. Klimas, et al. 1985. Mothers of infants with the acquired immunodeficiency syndrome. *JAMA* 255:363–66.

Shaw, N. 1985. *California models for women's AIDS education and services.* San Francisco: AIDS Foundation.

Stewart, G. J., J. P. P. Tyler, G. L. Cunningham, et al. 1985. Transmission of human T-cell lymphotropic virus type III (HTLV-III) by artificial insemination by donor. *Lancet* 2:581–84.

Wofsy, C., J. Cohen, L. B. Hauer, et al. 1986. Isolation of HTLV-III/LAV from cervical secretions of women at risk for AIDS. *Lancet* 1:527–29.

Wykoff, R. F. 1986. Letter to the editor. *JAMA* 255:1704–5.

Ziegler, J. B., D. A. Cooper, R. O. Johnson, et al. 1985. Postnatal transmission of AIDs-associated retrovirus from mother to infant. *Lancet* 1:896–98.

16

Substance Abuse as a Cofactor for AIDS

BARBARA G. FALTZ AND SCOTT MADOVER

It becomes apparent when we look at the connection between substance abuse and AIDS that they are linked in five ways.

The first and most obvious link is the direct transmission of the
AIDS virus through the sharing of hypodermic needles, syringes, and
paraphernalia used in "shooting up" drugs. According to the CDC, IV
use is the primary risk factor for 17 percent of persons with AIDS. In
addition, 11 percent of the gay and bisexual men report a history of IV
drug use, making a total of 28 percent of those with AIDS IV drug
users (CDC 1985).

The second link of substance abuse with AIDS is the transmission of
the virus by infected IV drug users to their sexual partners in either
heterosexual or homosexual contact. Of those reported cases of heterosexual transmission of the disease in the United States, the overwhelming preponderance has been in women (CDC 1985).

Third, infected women who are IV drug users or who are sexual
partners of IV drug users can transmit the virus during the neonatal
period.

In cohort studies, a correlation between the use of volatile amyl and
butyl nitrites (poppers) and the development of KS has been demonstrated (Newell et al. 1985). Although they are not directly linked to
AIDS, alcohol, marijuana, cocaine, and amphetamines have been
demonstrated to be immunosuppressant. We feel that persons who
have been exposed to the AIDS virus by their sexual partners or
through IV drug use need to reexamine their use of immunosuppressant drugs—particularly their use of poppers.

Finally, there is the factor of increased sexual and needle-using behavior while under the influence of alcohol or drugs. In a report prepared for the San Francisco AIDS Foundation, the Research and Decisions Corporation (1985) cited the following findings:

The results suggest that there is a significant problem with drug use among the city's self-identifying gay and bisexual male population and that this problem may be perpetrating the AIDS epidemic. When asked if they were ever high or drunk while having sex, nearly one in five (18 percent) say they are at least so intoxicated that they would not want to drive a car. Fourteen percent say [that] they have used IV drugs at some point in their lives. Just 3 percent report doing so in the past six months, but this 3 percent accounts for 38 percent of all anal intercourse and 48 percent of all fisting with nonprimary partners. . . . This strong association between IV drug use and these unsafe sex practices suggests that . . . the AIDS education issue cannot be separated from the larger issue of drug abuse.

In addition, the report noted the significant finding that "61 percent agree that they are more likely to have unsafe sex when using alcohol or drugs."

The myth that AIDS is a gay white male disease is particularly fallacious when we talk about the substance abuse and AIDS link. Half of the IV drug abusers with AIDS are black, more than a quarter are Hispanic, and fewer than 20 percent are Caucasian. More than half of the women with AIDS are IV drug users. This myth can have predictable deleterious effects on the planning of prevention and treatment strategies for IV drug abusers. The myth can also serve to bolster the denial of nonwhite addicts that they need to be concerned about AIDS. A strategy for AIDS prevention among needle users must be responsive to the real demographics of the epidemic.

The five linking factors discussed above make it essential to have substance abuse evaluation of clients in risk groups for AIDS. This includes persons who are seropositive for the AIDS antibody, who have ARC, or who have AIDS. The evaluation should determine the kind and frequency of substances used, and specific inquiry must be made into IV drug use.

In our substance abuse assessments we ask about current medical problems in addition to details about any AIDS-related diagnosis. A thorough drug and alcohol history covering length and patterns of use and last use is obtained. We particularly look for the following indications of addiction:

1. Preoccupation with the drug(s) of choice or alcohol;
2. drinking or drug use while alone;
3. rapid intake of the substance (for example, gulping drinks);
4. self-medication for anxiety or sadness with alcohol or drugs;

5. attempts to protect one's supply by hiding drugs or buying extra in anticipation of projected need;
6. loss of control of amount or frequency of use (e.g., drinking ten instead of two drinks as originally planned);
7. increased tolerance (for example, using more than other people without obvious intoxication);
8. blackouts;
9. withdrawal symptoms.

After long-term use or intense short-term use, people often experience numerous emotional, social, vocational, legal, and financial problems. We assess the extent and severity of these consequences. Our working definition of addiction is that if problems such as those discussed occur as a result of drug or alcohol use *and* the person continues to use them, an addiction is present.

After the assessment, we share our findings with the clients and educate them as to the nature of the disease of alcoholism/chemical dependency and its progression. We relate the problems uncovered to the use of drugs and alcohol. We confront rationalizations, minimization, and denial of substance abuse if they exist. We make recommendations and referrals based upon clients' willingness to examine their addiction and their motivation for treatment.

We also discuss the relationship between AIDS and substance abuse, and what can be done to minimize the risks of contracting AIDS. We cover the AIDS risk-reduction behaviors found in the following checklist:

IF YOU DON'T WANT TO GET AIDS . . .
1. THE BEST WAY IS TO QUIT SHOOTING UP DRUGS:
   · You can get help to stop.
2. IF YOU MUST SHOOT UP:
   · Don't share needles.
   · You can get AIDS by sharing a needle or syringe.
   · Remember that people can look healthy and still carry the AIDS virus.
3. CLEAN YOUR WORKS:
   · Flush needle and syringe with Clorox bleach. Rinse well with water.
   · Or boil for 15 minutes.

4. USE OF OTHER DRUGS:
   - Remember that alcohol, marijuana, speed, cocaine, and "poppers" can lower your resistance.
5. REDUCE RISK OF GETTING AIDS SEXUALLY:
   - Use condoms.
   - Avoid contact with semen (come) or blood.
   - See safe sex guidelines.
   - Remember that people can look healthy and still carry the AIDS virus.
   - Having sex while "loaded" can increase your possibility of taking sexual risks due to impaired judgment.
6. WANT MORE INFORMATION???
   - DRUG HOTLINE* (415) 752-3400

Often, physicians and other health care workers have difficulty in diagnosing and treating substance abuse disorders in persons diagnosed as having AIDS. The issue of AIDS and substance abuse raises critical clinical, ethical, and personal concerns for medical and mental health professionals. In order to provide quality care for all persons with AIDS, the following issues must be addressed.

Why bother?   Concerns are often expressed that the patient will die anyway, that substance abuse treatment will take away a "coping mechanism," that treatment is strenuous and confrontive and will increase stress, and that it is a question of a patient's free choice to use or not. In other words, "Why bother initiating substance abuse treatment?"

This question addresses the basic issue of the quality of life possible after diagnosis of a life-threatening illness. For an individual troubled by the chaotic life-style often accompanying active drug or alcohol abuse, the crisis of the AIDS diagnosis may generate a willingness to examine the primary question, "What will I do with the rest of my life?" One client chose to begin treatment after discussing his situation because, as he stated, "I don't want to die drunk the way my father did." A client may choose to continue using drugs, even at the risk of jeopardizing assistance with housing or other services. In either event, the choice to seek treatment and growth or to remain addicted should be made by the client. What we hope is that health care providers rec-

*Every locality should use nearest available hotline numbers.

ognize the need for this choice and facilitate exposure to substance abuse evaluation.

Substance Abuse as a "Moral Issue."   Often substance abuse is viewed as a weakness or a choice—not as a disease. A person with this view may feel that treatment should consist of a lecture on "right" or "wrong" behavior and/or an exhortation to control one's impulses. Unfortunately, neither action will lead to a lasting elimination of the problem.

Substance abuse is a disease characterized by the inability of a person to control the amount or frequency of alcohol or drug use. It "involves the whole person, physically, mentally, psychologically, and spiritually. The most significant characteristics of the disease are that it is primary, progressive, chronic, and fatal" (Johnson 1980). There is hope, however, that it can be arrested with treatment and a continuing recovery program such as Alcoholics or Narcotics Anonymous. If it is viewed as a question of morality or "will power," treatment will be aborted and the addiction process will progress.

Anxiety.   Many obvious and some more subtle anxieties are associated with the confrontation of substance abuse problems in a person with AIDS. Again, practitioners may fear that the patient will experience additional stress or deprivation resulting in increased emotional difficulties. A fear of alienating a patient in his/her time of need results in anticipated guilt. In general, a tendency to minimize confrontation arises from a fear that a person with AIDS is fragile in *all* areas and needs extra protection. A careful look at one's own anxieties in connection with working with the complex problems associated with the diagnosis of both AIDS/ARC and substance abuse is essential.

Confusion About Appropriate Interventions for Denial.   It is appropriate for a person grieving about the diagnosis of a life-threatening illness to deny that this threat is real. This type of denial is usually supported until a person can begin to absorb the impact of the implications of diagnosis. In the case of substance abuse, however, denial is the chief defense against seeing the extent of the problem and the consequences of the addiction. It prevents a person from seeking treatment for alcoholism or chemical dependency for which there is hope of remission.

It is, therefore, important to time substance abuse interventions carefully. The most productive time to address this concern is after a client is becoming more accepting of the AIDS diagnosis. It is not appropriate to intervene while a client is still actively denying the presence of the disease. Helpful interventions dealing with denial and other behavioral manifestations of addiction are discussed below.

Manifestations of Addiction.   Dealing with many behavioral manifestations of addiction is often frustrating. Manipulative behaviors are often part of this picture. Flattery, intrusiveness, intimidation, inflammatory remarks, and bargaining are common. Attempts may be made to turn other clients against staff or agencies with such comments as "You know what *they* did to me?" or "You're not like the others at the clinic, you understand me." A client may appear overly helpless or compliant or, conversely, may repeatedly question the staff's actions. In addition to the denial or minimization of a substance abuse problem, there is often concurrent justification and rationalization of it and other actions such as "If you had my situation, you'd drink too!" A client may be evasive or avoid contact altogether, perhaps fearing confrontation.

Each of these behaviors assures the client of protection of the continued use and abuse of drugs or alcohol by the attempt to avoid confrontation, deflection of attention, justification of continued use secondary to staff rejection, and the like.

One particular blind alley that can entice a health care worker is a client's admission of a substance abuse problem coupled with the invitation to help search for the answer to the question "Why do I drink so much?" Insight therapy may be helpful in many areas, but insight is not the immediate goal of treatment for addiction. The truth is that a person who is addicted to alcohol or drugs uses them because he *cannot* control their use, regardless of life's circumstances.

The following are guidelines to successful intervention with the behaviors associated with active addiction:

1. Encourage constructive expression of feelings and listen.
2. Express caring and concern for the individual.
3. Hold the individual responsible for his/her actions.
4. Ensure that there are consistent consequences for negative behaviors.
5. Talk to the individual about specific actions that are disruptive or disturbing.
6. Don't compromise your own values or expectations.
7. Communicate your plan of action to other relevant staff members.
8. Monitor your own reactions to client's behavior for possible interference with the treatment relationship.

In addition, it is important to avoid interactions like those listed below in treating substance abuse:

1. Minimizing or not talking about abuse or the results of it.
2. Avoiding confrontation.
3. Making excuses for continuing drug or alcohol use.
4. Saving the client from feeling the results of his/her addiction.
5. Trying to "protect" the client from alcohol or drugs.
6. Viewing alcoholism or addiction as a weakness rather than an illness.
7. Trying to find the cause, hoping that the disease will go away when the cause is found.
8. Encouraging the use of "will power" or other oversimplified "cures."
9. Expressing anger, frustration, blame, or disappointment toward the client who continues to use drugs or alcohol.
10. Gossiping about the client to others.

Priority issues.   So many other physical, emotional, financial, and legal concerns are associated with AIDS that often substance abuse problems are not seen as a priority to be addressed as aggressively as some other needs.

Minimizing or ignoring this aspect of the treatment picture can cause a major problem. It can impede progress in other areas. Financial assistance may be used to purchase drugs, and physical, emotional, legal problems may be exacerbated.

Motivation.   People who are actively pursuing their addiction feel little motivation for treatment. Many of those who are diagnosed with AIDS have not felt the continued painful consequences of years of drinking or drug use, such as loss of relationships and employment, legal or financial difficulties, other physical problems. They or health care workers may not feel that the problem "is bad enough yet" to seek treatment.

In situations with limited motivation for treatment, it is important to educate clients about the consequences to themselves and others of continued use of immunosuppressant drugs, of unsafe needle sharing and sexual practices. Even if this does not result in changed behavior, it will serve to remove the alibi of "I didn't know" viz-a-viz the connection of AIDS with substance abuse.

As the epidemic has unfolded, a growing relationship between it and substance abuse has evolved. In San Francisco, a task force of service providers from the substance abuse community and members of existing AIDS agencies met to discuss the need for additional services for those affected by the dual problems of AIDS and substance abuse. Through discussions with the San Francisco Department of Public

Health and the Community Substance Abuse Services, the AIDS Substance Abuse program of the University of California, San Francisco, AIDS Health Project was developed. In February 1985, the AIDS Substance Abuse program began to offer the following services: consultation about drug and alcohol concerns for persons with AIDS; support groups for those with AIDS or ARC who are in recovery from alcoholism/chemical dependency; education and consultation for health care and substance abuse agencies; public education about AIDS and substance abuse.

Clinical issues have been sharpened as a result of this experience. Clients were referred by substance abuse or AIDS care delivery agencies. Eighty percent of them were diagnosed with either AIDS or ARC; 58 percent reported regular needle use; many were polydrug abusers; the major substances abused were alcohol (55 percent), amphetamines (44 percent), and opiates (22 percent).

As the AIDS epidemic progresses, the need to address substance abuse issues will intensify. Developing assessment procedures that combine knowledge of both areas and providing professional education to health care workers have already enhanced communitywide discussion of the issues.

References

Centers for Infectious Diseases, Centers for Disease Control. 1985. *Acquired immunodeficiency syndrome (AIDS) weekly surveillance report—United States AIDS activity*. November 18.

Johnson, V. 1980. *I'll quit tomorrow*. San Francisco: Harper & Row.

Newell, G. R. et al. 1985. Risk factor analysis among men referred for possible acquired immune deficiency syndrome. *Preven Med* 14:81–91.

Research and Decisions Corp. 1985. A report on designing an effective AIDS prevention campaign strategy for San Francisco: Results from the second probability sample of an urban gay male community. San Francisco AIDS Foundation. Typescript.

17

Counseling Survivors

PAUL SHEARER AND LEON MCKUSICK

Many theorists and clinicians have provided us with exemplary discussion of the grief process and effective means of treatment (Becker
1973, Levine 1982, 1984, Prakes 1974). Perhaps the most well known is
Elisabeth Kubler-Ross (1969), who originally described five stages of
grief—denial, bargaining, anger, depression, and acceptance. Others
have challenged the concreteness of these as stages and have suggested
that the five concepts be viewed as psychological attributes of a bereavement process or an adjustment to a life-threatening event, especially to death. Thus, as we interpret the phenomenon of grief in the
AIDS epidemic we will discuss how these five forces are at work in the
instances of surviving family and lovers who sustained losses in the
AIDS epidemic.

Family Grief in AIDS

One of the new genre of not so funny AIDS jokes places the gay man
in front of his parents with good news and bad news: the bad news
first being that the son is gay, the good news that he is dying of AIDS.
Certainly these jokes reflect the stigmatizing nature of society's attitudes toward homosexuality and, by association, toward AIDS. This
one makes fun of the double adjustment that families have to undergo
in coping with a son who has AIDS in those unfortunate cases where
two facts are forced into their awareness at the same time—which can
create an immense conflict and trauma for parents. The level of denial
in such families is probably fairly high to begin with if the sexual identity of the son is undisclosed before the diagnosis. Thus, the task of the
family therapist includes helping parents to confront the psychological
pain caused by the loss of this defense.

In many cases, once these conflicts are resolved, parents can approach the son with more love and support and stay close through the illness, which substantially changes the fabric of the relationship, as well as relationships throughout the family. One man described sitting with his mother for two hours after he told her of his diagnosis of KS. She wanted others in the close extended family network not to know about his disease, fearing stigmatization. His argument persisted. It was important to his health that he be supported by all who loved him. Finally, she relented. He discovered when he told his uncles, aunts, and cousins that all of them already knew about his homosexuality. Indeed, they also had been concerned about his mother over the years and would have lent her more emotional support had they not tacitly agreed to her conspiracy of silence.

Any painful event is better dealt with if held in the light and not hidden away. Grief that becomes protracted has a secretive and depressing but special and private flavor, which usually dissipates when someone else is brought into the grief process. Thus, this mother, who resolved her denial by throwing a large party in his community to celebrate her son's fortieth birthday with all his friends, moved closer to him and found a much more profound experience for herself, despite the painful confrontation.

Many men, after leaving the family home, develop a new "chosen family" of significant friends. These chosen families usually rally to the bedside of the person with AIDS with social, financial, and life management support. In a smooth process after death, this network and the nuclear family can share their ritual grieving together. One mother, after having come from the Midwest to her son's community for his memorial service, looked out from the podium at the sea of faces of his friends and said, "It certainly proves the feeling I've had for years that my son was loved and lovable to be here among his friends and to feel the love and support you have shown me this week."

In some cases, however, families do not cross these boundaries, creating ritual and personal grief processes that exclude friends of the gay man. Whereas this honors the philosophical or spiritual needs of the family, it may also be alienating. One man had to sit behind the sanctuary, with a wall between him and his companion's coffin during the memorial service, which had been closed to everyone but "immediate family." The two men had been constant companions for fifteen years and had shared everything, but the survivor found that he had no sanctions, social or legal. He also was denied bereavement leave by his employer. If the family does not recognize the viability of their gay son's lifestyle or the rights of his chosen partner to grief or to decisions regarding the estate, conflict can result. The situation is often extremely volatile, given the stress of all involved as well as the emotional and financial stakes. It may be necessary at this time for a therapist to mediate conflicts and, if alleviating confrontation, smooth the transitional process and cushion feelings of anger and guilt in the family.

Like war, AIDS is stealing young people from their families. One mother confided, "It's not supposed to happen this way, he was supposed to bury me!" She grew angry, furious that first she buried her parents and now her son. Soon after the anger came the guilt, ridiculing herself for somehow not being able to save him. She was solid as a rock throughout his illness, kindly fending off support for fear it would break her. Then, after he died, she no longer had to be strong and she talked about her own concerns. "I'm not sure how I'll talk to people back home about this—they're all so scared to death of AIDS. In fact, I was too until he got sick, then I lost my own fear." Becoming closer to a dying son may awaken one's own reactions to the approach of death. There is a profound wisdom to be learned by families who do suffer this loss, if helped by the compassionate clinician to integrate the experience.

Counseling Bereaved Lovers

When two people who love each other are separated by the death of one, the survivor normally becomes host to a number of confusing thoughts and feelings that ebb and flow without apparent predictability. Certainly, there is grief, one of life's more profound emotional experiences, but also celebration and solace that the dying is over. Characteristically, there are loneliness, memories, and heartache. It is a time of transition, when one reassesses his beliefs and his relationship to the rest of the world. During this sensitive time the survivor can expect to feel tearful, angry at the least provocation, misunderstood by those who have not also suffered loss, or even guilty for no good reason.

A great majority of survivors of lovers who died from AIDS are young people who have not before experienced mortal loss, making their pain all the more confusing. Many of the grieved are youths and their deaths seemingly senseless. It is not uncommon to hear the bereaved say, "I am going crazy." The clinician can offer simple validation of the bizarre nature of his client's experience with the reassurance that, yes, it is an enormous tragedy to lose a loved one to AIDS.

During clinical work with six surviving male lovers of men who died from AIDS, common characteristics were found that may be helpful to a clinician approaching treatment of bereavement in gay men.

First, these men were experiencing the stages of bereavement in a community that is itself becoming expert in the stages of bereavement, including denial. Each man seen for bereavement counseling complained that his friends were getting tired of hearing him talk about his lover. All described pressure from their associates to conduct their grief in various appropriate fashions. From a close female friend: "It's been three months. I think it is time you gave away Tommy's clothes." From a café acquaintance, whom AIDS had made an expert in matters of departed spirits: "How can you continue to imprison your lover's soul by wishing he was still beside you. I implore you. Let him go. He has much more important things to do."

At the beginning of therapy with these men, it was necessary to encourage them to use however much time they needed to talk about, think about, have erotic fantasies about, or cry about the loss of their loves, exclusive of any schedule. This permission alone assists the process, because it counteracts whatever need the gay man's friends may have (or pressure he may feel from his peers) to bury the process of bereavement soon after the funeral.

After the death, the lover may become much more immediately aware of his own possible susceptibility to AIDS, a contagion fear that he had suspended in order to remain close to his dying friend now coming back strongly. Moreover, he is acutely aware of what AIDS looks like and can be petrified of getting it from or giving it to anyone else. Consequently, sexual repression and anxiety attacks about contagion occurred in the men treated.

Like all specters, that of AIDS is mysterious and therefore frightening; society at large does not want to be touched by it. Thus, the survivor can often feel stigmatized by his association with the victim. On becoming aware that he is HIV seropositive, one man expressed guilt that he had possibly transmitted AIDS to his lover. Simple extension of understanding and compassion can help here to soften feelings of leprous alienation or the person's horror of his own contagiousness. Since the disease kept them on exhausting schedules before their lovers' death, these men have also been too busy to worry about dating and safe sex and may need good motherly advice at this time, reassurances that they are capable of being close to men physically without exposure to or transmission of the AIDS virus.

In this instance, denial may lend some saving grace. Interestingly, in this small sample of men in psychotherapy, those adapt psychologically more quickly who deny causality between their lovers' illness and their own susceptibility to AIDS. They are less likely to become symbiotically depressed, less likely to long suicidally for their lovers; they are more likely to become engaged in new relationships and less likely to have fears about contamination, even while being cautious about transmission. In this population, research results that link bereavement and depression to suppression of immune function are particularly relevant (Bartrop et al. 1977, Schleifer et al. 1983). For the therapist, the question arises of how much depression and dysphoria should be encouraged as clients work through feelings about their lovers' death. This is a dynamic question that usually must be related to each individual's coping styles and personality factors. Fortunately, it is most often answered by the client himself as he naturally moves between the constituent phases of denial and acceptance.

Those who were primarily responsible for the day-to-day care of their lovers have a much more difficult time emotionally, particularly if they had conflicts about the care with their lovers' families. These men are caught in a stance of protective vigilance at the moment of their lovers' death from which it is very difficult to relax—in one case for two years after the death. Gay lovers often have to fight the family for legitimacy, and then for primacy of their bond and the independence of their relationship. In the case of AIDS, however, this fight may take place over the hospital bed at a time when the spoils of victory for the already embattled lover become the right to embrace and care for a man in his dying hours.

Lovers are universally idealized, particularly in the early stages of the relationship. A rigid idealization of the dead lover can occur, making new boyfriends unwelcome. At the same time that each of our bereaved patients has longed for the closeness and support he gave his dying partner, he has also compared anyone who approaches him with the idealized image of his partner, thus heightening his loneliness for a time. In the last stages of his life, the person with AIDS and his lover return to what Mattison and McWhirter in their book *The Male Couple* (1984) call stage one or the blending stage, where romance is extremely high and ego boundaries are just as loose. The only problem is that then the lover dies and leaves behind a fiercely devoted widower. This patient's dream came six months after his lover's death:

> There was Joe in the bedroom. He was weak and skinny. We hugged and kissed (not on the mouth) and cried, joy and anguish. Joe needed to put on the white pajamas I bought for him at Neiman Marcus. He needed me to brace and support him while putting on the tops. We glanced in a

mirror together. He looked bad and was bent over. Then he hung with his arms around my neck and shoulders while I walked into the other rooms, looking for the bottoms. I told him in tears how good it felt to be touched and touch after so long. We stood embracing in the front room face to face and crying as we were merged there together.

There is a hidden asset in this psychologically painful epidemic. These men have experienced many of the necessary ingredients of love: devotion, putting the other person first, seeing the best of oneself in the other. As most relationships progress, a working balance of autonomy and dependence is negotiated and maintained. Because of the inordinate dependence of those suffering from terminal AIDS, the youthfulness of the men it attacks, and the untimely interruption to intimacy that a lover's death brings, he who is left behind has sacrificed his autonomy and needs to regain it. Unlike a relationship that ends because of incompatibility, here it is difficult to mobilize anger at the departed partner as a means of recovering one's sense of well-being and rightness.

In the special instance of bereavement, the therapist can help the partner finish the dialogue of the relationship and prepare to move on. When a persistently depressed griever confessed in a session that he had private conversations daily with his dead lover, some of them about the therapy and the therapist, the perspective of the deceased was invited into treatment, through the use of a gestalt type of dialogue. After that invitation, the three—therapist, client, and the man's lost lover—moved much more quickly and less painfully until the client was willing at a later date to assimilate his lost lover's opinions and impressions as his own. Perhaps not so coincidentally, as this man accepted his lover's death, he was also able to accept another man into his life as a primary dating partner, and the new relationship began developing into a more substantial and connected partnership. He noted that he felt his lost partner's approval and support for his new happiness.

Finally, after their lovers have died, those who involve themselves in AIDS volunteer activity recover more quickly. These days, if one does not withdraw but looks around, one can see a universal human phenomenon occurring. Having already had a crash course in being helpers and care-givers, these men may do well if encouraged to become involved with an AIDS volunteer organization. Within these organizations they also may find new friends who have similar stories to tell. Since the loss of friends and lovers to AIDS has increasingly become a communitywide occurrence, a great deal of wisdom and support is available alongside the great deal of pain the community is experiencing.

References

Bartrop, R. W., L. Lazarus, E. Luckherst, et al. 1977. Depressed lymphocyte function after bereavement. *Lancet* 1:834–36.

Becker, E. 1973. *The denial of death.* New York: Free Press.

Kubler-Ross, E. 1969. *On death and dying.* New York: Macmillan.

Levine, S. 1984. *Meetings at the edge.* Garden City, N.Y.: Anchor Books.

———. 1982. *Who dies.* Garden City: Anchor Books.

Mattison, A. M., and D. P. McWhirter. 1984. *The male couple.* Englewood Cliffs, N.J.: Prentice-Hall.

Prakes, C. 1974. *Bereavement.* New York: International Universities Press.

Schleifer, S. J., S. E. Keller, et al. 1983. Suppression of lymphocyte stimulation following bereavement. *JAMA* 250 (3):374–77.

PART IV

Public Health Issues

18

Psychosocial Sensitivity in Hospital Care: San Francisco General Hospital

PAUL VOLBERDING, GAYLING GEE, BROOKS LINTON

Paul Volberding: A model system for the care of patients with AIDS has been developed that recognizes the many medical, psychological, and societal difficulties involved. This model emphasizes multidisciplinary medical and psychosocial care equally. An effective system must recognize the complexities in both areas and have staff and facilities able to provide necessary services. A third component is the integration of inpatient and outpatient functions.

The care of patients requires several medical specialties. Oncologists and infectious disease experts are fundamental. Also important are specialists in those organ systems that are particularly affected by the disease, including pulmonary physicians, neurologists, neurosurgeons, dermatologists, ophthalmologists, and radiation therapists, as well as many others.

Whereas most medical centers have specialists in each of these areas, patient access to and communication among these services may be problems. Unless the specialists are familiar with AIDS and are readily available, care will be compromised. For this reason, multidisciplinary AIDS clinics are strongly recommended. In such clinics, most clinical problems can be addressed, reducing miscommunication and improving patient convenience and compliance. Also, larger multidisciplinary clinics are capable of providing more complex outpatient management (for example, medications by central line) and substantial cost savings may be realized by the clinics in limiting the necessity for expensive inpatient care.

Editor's note: This article combines the contributions of three authors from San Francisco General Hospital to present the patient's world from three perspectives: medicine, nursing, and social work. In this manner, psychosocial aspects of AIDS treatment are thoroughly explored.

Multidisciplinary AIDS clinics should include, at a minimum, representatives from psychiatry and medical social work to deal with the common, often severe psychosocial problems and financial difficulties of patients with AIDS. Community organizations, which can provide extremely important services, should be invited to participate as an integral part of clinic structures.

Outpatient management must be the desired goal of care, both to allow the patient as much time as possible at home and to reduce overall costs. Approaching this goal, however, will result in an increase in the severity of disease in outpatients. Although this emphasis on outpatient management will limit the need for hospitalizing patients, those patients who do then require hospitalization will be extremely ill.

Complex outpatient management requires rigorous planning and close integration with inpatient services. Patients leaving the hospital may require immediate care from several community agencies as well as frequent outpatient clinic visits. Management plans such as these must be cautiously designed and instituted before the patient is discharged from the hospital, and they must be carefully monitored after the patient is discharged. Otherwise, frequent and avoidable readmissions will occur. Maximum cooperation and communication between outpatient and inpatient staffs are facilitated by integrated AIDS clinics and outpatient units.

The San Francisco General Hospital is a large public hospital owned by the City and County of San Francisco and staffed by the University of California, San Francisco. In January 1983 a multidisciplinary AIDS outpatient clinic opened with attending staff from the medical oncology and infectious disease divisions. From the first, this clinic also included medical social workers and representatives from community support agencies. Also in 1983, the first AIDS inpatient unit in the country was formed at the hospital. Patients with AIDS are admitted to this unit under the care of general medical service teams composed of attending staff, medical house staff, and medical students. Cooperation in patient management promotes the development of consistent philosophies of care.

The AIDS inpatient unit at the hospital opened in July 1983 to ensure comprehensive and sensitive patient care by a centralized nursing staff. Although there was serious concern that such a unit could increase the isolation and stigmatization of AIDS patients, the opposite has occurred: The AIDS inpatient unit is widely perceived as a near-ideal place in which to be treated—because of both its state-of-the-art medical care and its expert nursing. Several factors have contributed to this success. First, all members of the nursing staff volunteered to work with patients with AIDS. Second, no barriers were erected to isolate the unit from the rest of the hospital. Finally, the gay community was invited to participate in the unit's development, thus increasing open communication and a sense of mutual trust.

The nursing staff of both the AIDS clinic and the inpatient unit has rapidly become expert in AIDS-related medical and psychosocial issues. Patients in both areas have immediate access to current information about AIDS and about available community services. Patients newly diagnosed with the syndrome are offered intensive education about their disease and what they can anticipate during their clinical course. Crisis intervention can be delivered immediately after identification of emotional problems. Because much of the counseling is done by nursing and psychosocial support staff, burdens on house staff are somewhat eased. A final benefit is the management of media access to patients. Medical and nursing staff are able to help ensure that the message relayed by the media concerning AIDS is accurate and educational rather than sensational and alarmist.

Although the system of health care we have evolved works extremely well in our community and facility, not all elements of the system will be possible or desirable in other settings. Among factors limiting the application of this system are the number of patients seen and the resources available. Because the start-up costs for establishing a multidisciplinary AIDS service are considerable, there must be a large number of patients with AIDS. Hospitals caring for small numbers of patients may be able to incorporate required services effectively into existing systems. Where patients with AIDS are more numerous, coordinated services producing fewer and briefer hospitalizations may be cost-effective.

A second factor limiting the provision of dedicated services in hospitals is the fear—sometimes stated openly, other times covertly—that hospitals providing coordinated AIDS services will be seen by the public as "AIDS hospitals." In the case of private facilities, the concern is that this label may discourage referral of patients with other illnesses and result in major financial losses.

It is a challenge for hospitals to provide comprehensive, sensitive care for patients with AIDS. The system of care should not increase the suffering of the patients. Whereas not every hospital can be expected to make a commitment to provide comprehensive care, more should be encouraged to do so. All hospitals caring for patients must recognize and address the clinical variability of the manifestations, the multisystem nature of the disease, the intensity and complexity of therapy, and the profound psychosocial consequences of the disease.

Gayling Gee: When I first started working with the oncology service at San Francisco General Hospital in 1981, I was the only nurse there, hired by Paul Volberding, the newly appointed chief of medical oncology, to help him develop services in what was a single, half-day-a-week oncology clinic. An average outpatient clinic for us consisted of about eighteen patients.

That summer, in 1981, we saw one Kaposi's sarcoma patient. He was a twenty-one-year-old gay male prostitute who had early KS that was rapidly progressing. He had a dependent personality, and he would show up at clinic in the morning. The clerks who let him in were kind enough to let him stay in our conference room. I would find him there some mornings, and he would say, "Oh, Gayling. I don't know what to do. I'm so—everything's just gone wrong." Because he had been so ill, he was no longer able to earn a living and he seemed quite isolated. He had extensive lesions on his skin, his legs, his arms, his face; internally, he had KS in his lungs, esophagus, all the way down his bowel system, in his liver, in his brain. Imagine how devastating the disease was for him! He was, I believe, from West Virginia, and his family had basically disowned him. He died in Intensive Care, primarily from KS in his lung. Sadly, the way he lived the last few months was really the way he died. No one was there to claim the body. It took several weeks before a sister finally came out to take the body back to his home for burial.

What strikes me now when I talk about services for AIDS patients is that then, in 1981, we had no services to offer him. The Medical Social Service Department was just beginning to figure out what AIDS was and how difficult it was for people with AIDS to gain access to the social services system. There was no one to help him and to be with him at the very last.

Within five years, I became head nurse of a combined AIDS and Oncology Clinic, Ward 86. We developed six AIDS clinics and two oncology clinics. And we are expanding into more AIDS clinics because we are getting more space on our unit. Instead of one KS patient visit a week, we now average about 250 AIDS-related encounters per week. In the fiscal year 1983–84 we had about 3,600 encounters; in the fiscal year 1984–85 our clinic had 12,000 encounters. That is a 300 percent increase. And each AIDS case we see now is very complicated.

From one nurse and one doctor, the clinic staff has grown to include one administrative head nurse, three nurse practitioners, four staff nurses, one LVN, two phlebotomists, five clerical staff members, one clinical pharmacist, four protocol managers, and six attending physicians. And we also have added to the number of physicians who rotate through our clinic.

The clinics we have now include two general AIDS clinics on Monday morning and afternoon and an AIDS/ARC clinic on Tuesday morning where the focus is lymphadenopathy syndrome and ARC. We now have two oncology clinics. We also have one nurse-screening clinic on Thursday morning, in which patients are screened and evaluated for AIDS. We have a Thursday afternoon AIDS opportunistic infection clinic, and a Friday morning AIDS/KS clinic. The clinics are basically open Monday through Friday, and all categories are seen—from "Worried Well" through those who are dying. There is sufficient overlapping of staff among the clinics for patients to transfer from one to another with minimal interruption of care.

San Francisco General Hospital is unique in having both an outpatient AIDS clinic and an inpatient AIDS unit, 5B. When a patient needs to be admitted, Ward 5B is checked first for available beds. In 1983, the first six months were rather easy. Members of the 5B staff were often being asked to rotate off the unit because not all the beds were filled. That is not a problem now. There is a long waiting list of AIDS patients, many who have to be hospitalized on other units. Connection with those AIDS patients is maintained by nurses and by the Shanti counselors (see below) on 5B.

Services provided by our clinic nursing staff include outpatient chemotherapy administration, outpatient blood transfusions, central line care, and clinical research. We have done and are doing several experimental studies, in which many of our patients are involved. Our standards of care follow directly upon the results of these studies.

Because AIDS patients along the entire spectrum of the disease process are followed in the clinic, our model of care must be flexible enough to accommodate most needs. From the initial screening and evaluation through the diagnosis, the patient regards us as his primary care provider. We see him through clinical remissions, progression, numerous experimental treatment protocols, and, sadly, terminal care.

In addition to a full complement of medical and nursing staff, the outpatient clinic also has three very important integrated psychosocial components. The first one is the Shanti Project: The Shanti counselor provides emotional support and crisis counseling for every AIDS patient in the clinic. The Shanti volunteer practical support staff of six helps us with a thousand and one things to which the nursing staff cannot always devote time—making runs to the pharmacy to drop off prescriptions for the patients so that the typical two-to-three-hour wait at our county hospital pharmacy is shortened, escorting patients to the hospital to get a chest X-ray, or even just waiting with a patient at the front door for a cab. Shanti volunteers help us enormously in both the AIDS outpatient clinic and on the AIDS inpatient unit, facilitating patient access to these services. The Shanti Project also has an ongoing series of support groups for patients and their friends. The AIDS Health Project has provided us with a clinic-based psychiatric social worker, who works with patients on crisis issues as well as chronic emotional issues. The Medical Social Service Department of San Francisco General Hospital also has recognized the needs of AIDS patients in the clinic and has assigned a full-time medical social worker to help the AIDS patients in the clinic with such concrete needs as disability, housing, transportation, and food.* This explains how we deliver AIDS care in terms of organization, but how does this translate into the human, emotional aspects of what we do?

Working with AIDS means that we become totally involved with people and with AIDS care. The clinic staff is a very tight, cohesive group. We have our share of burnout, which is cyclical; everybody goes up and down. It's bad when everyone is down at the same time, but mostly it's fifty-fifty, fortunately, with half of us up and half of us down. We have our share of acting out, of grieving, of running into an empty room and just crying, because we have been so involved with a patient who finally seems not able to recover. But the other side of that is that we care an awful lot about one another. We take good care of one another. If we find that one or the other of us is not doing so well, someone will take that person aside and say, "What's going on? Let me know." If that's your time to cry, that's your time to cry. We play together, we party together. We have our share of Christmas parties, birthday parties, showers, and other celebrations. I think the one thing that we still have, even though the average staff member now has worked in the clinic about two years, is a sense of humor. We are still able to laugh, and perhaps that's what keeps us going.

The other thing that really strikes me in AIDS care—and it is not just within our own clinic, but on Ward 5B, in Shanti, in the AIDS Foundation, in any AIDS agency we work with—and the one thing that really keeps us together is that we see patient care as a first priority. That cuts through any squabbles we may have either internally or with another organization. They are all temporary because we really perceive patient care as the reason for any of us to be here.

---

*Other community organizations are discussed at greater length below in Helen Schietinger, "Coordinated Community-Based AIDS Treatment."

Each of us in the clinic has had patients whom we remember best. Let me share with you reminiscences of some patients who really made an impact on me.

I knew a forty-four-year-old high school teacher who moved here from Michigan in August 1983 to get what he considered to be good AIDS care. We watched his progression from a few KS lesions on his skin when he first arrived to extensive lesions in May 1985. During those two years he was treated with a full gamut of what we had to offer. He received alpha interferon, gamma interferon, laser treatment, radiation therapy, and chemotherapy. His KS, which was so extensive, covered his skin with large purple lesions; they blocked his lymph nodes and caused extensive swelling in his legs and on his face, and it finally settled in his lungs. And that made him unable to breathe. He ultimately died in the hospital. He was anemic. Was it from his chronic illness or was it due to the KS involvement in his bone marrow? Was it a GI bleed in his gut from the KS there? He received several transfusions. He died in June 1985 after a very difficult last six months. He used to come into clinic and tell me, "Thank God you people are here. What would I ever do without you?" We gave him what I consider to be excellent care. It was the best AIDS care there was to give, and yet, in reality, we had nothing to offer him.

I also remember a thirty-one-year-old young man with KS, who was very bright, very brash. He loved to put us on the spot. If he could tease us, he would. There were no limits when he teased us. One would love him, but be helpless and nonplussed in the face of his banter. I saw him in the screening clinic in February 1983. He came in with his lover. He had a suspicious skin lesion, and we referred him to the hospital dermatology clinic for a biopsy. It turned out to be Kaposi's sarcoma. Within the next three months he and his lover ended their relationship. He too received the full range of the treatment options we had to offer. The KS spread to his lymph nodes, and his facial edema was quite severe. Often when he came into clinic, the edema would be so bad that his eyes would be swollen shut. His single lesion had spread to confluent purple lesions, and very often, from far away his face would look purple, not flesh-colored. On one occasion some high school girls wandered into the clinic and saw him sitting at the reception desk in his very advanced stage of KS. Frightened, they ran screaming down the hallway, leaving via the fire escape. There was really nothing we could do to shield him from this hurt. There he was, not feeling well, and so vulnerable, and there was someone screaming and running away from him because he looked so frightening. He also died in June 1985.

Both he and the teacher from Michigan were also taunted on the street and in buses by insensitive young people. A number of patients told me they were afraid to board a bus when school let out about three o'clock. If they saw teenagers that they thought were a little tough, they would not get on the bus, but wait for the next one.

I remember another twenty-six-year-old man, who always struck me as really being more of a boy. He had disseminated KS, with *Cryptosporidium* and chronic, persistent diarrhea. He was a very handsome young man who had modeled on the side. He was a weight lifter, proud of his muscles—his triceps and biceps—and his body generally. Initially, he would come into the clinic wearing his gym outfit with the leather belt tied around his waist. He would have his gamma interferon treatment and he would leave. We first saw him in December 1983. As it turned out, he had just one year to live. He went from 178 pounds to 130 pounds during that year. The last day he was in clinic he was too weak to stand long enough for us to weigh him. He died two weeks before Christmas with his mother and father at his bedside.

There is another side to what we see in the clinic. It's the side giving me hope that perhaps we can do something. I know another patient who is thirty-six years old, diagnosed with KS in May 1982. In August 1982 he began weekly chemotherapy treatments, which he received for two years. At the end of two years he was stable, with no evidence of tumor. And he is still healthy to date. This is the kind of case that I like to remind myself of.

Brookes Linton: Part of my job as medical social worker for Ward 5B, the AIDS inpatient unit at the San Francisco General Hospital, is to help coordinate the discharge planning for the patients there and for the AIDS patients on the other medical units in the hospital, except psychiatry. There are twelve beds on the unit, usually filled. The number of AIDS patients on other units in the hospital varies, as beds become vacant on the AIDS unit. Psychosocial issues receive excellent consideration from the professional and volunteer staffs on the inpatient unit. Three nurses take care of four patients each for twelve-hour shifts, which makes for very thorough, comprehensive care; in addition, an off-unit nurse sees all the AIDS and ARC patients elsewhere in the hospital, assessing their condition, determining priorities for transfer to 5B. Shanti counselors, in the hospital seven days a week, try to see all the AIDS patients.

My job has been to concentrate on the details of finances and the discharge planning, both of which are teamwork efforts that are usually interdependent and both emotional issues that require clearheaded arrangements. We try to find out as early as possible what the patients' financial and housing situations are and whether help will be needed in those areas at discharge time. The earlier plans can be made, the less anxiety patients have.

On Mondays, a discharge planning meeting is held with nurses, Shanti counselors, and staff, and also staff from the outside agencies. We are *extremely* fortunate in San Francisco to have such rich community resources developed to help with placement.

The average length of stay of an AIDS patient at San Francisco General is ten to twelve days. Recently I spoke with a social worker from a Washington, D.C., hospital, who had called to brainstorm about a particularly difficult placement problem she had: The patient was confused, no family, no friends. And she mentioned that the average length of stay for an AIDS patient in that hospital was seventy-one days. Such lengthy hospitalization indicates lack of outside resources.

Most patients do return to their original living situations, on their own, with lovers or friends, or with family. Those who cannot return to their living situations, however, need new housing or home care. For them, these resources have really been godsends.

Historically, I think that in San Francisco the first city government involvement began with a disturbance at the Jefferson Hotel in fall 1983. Jefferson is one of the hotels used by the city's Department of Social Services for its General Assistance recipients. And at the beginning of the AIDS crisis, AIDS patients on General Assistance were also being sent to the Jefferson, as we were following regular General Assistance procedure. When the other tenants found out, they objected strongly, because bathrooms were communal ones. This protest was strong impetus for some of the programs that were developed.

Basically, the programs we have access to for discharge planning are: (1) the emergency housing, free food bank, and financial and social services of the San Francisco AIDS Foundation; (2) residences managed by Shanti, and Shanti support services, both counseling and practical; (3) the AIDS Homecare program under Hospice; (4) three Bay Area Hospice facilities; (5) and some special agency programs: the AIDS Mental Health Project, the AIDS Fund, Visiting Nurse Association, Public Health nurses, substance abuse rehab programs, American Cancer Society, and the Department of Social Services itself.

Invaluable liaison people—one from Social Security and one from General Assistance—come to the hospital to fill out applications of patients directly.

Before Social Security allowed presumptive eligibility for AIDS patients and unless they were eligible for state disability, they had to live on General Assistance, which is now $288 a month plus food stamps, until SSI was processed, perhaps three to four months later. The Tenderloin in San Francisco is typical of the disreputable areas with affordable General Assistance hotels. Now SSI takes about three to four weeks to be processed.

The AIDS Foundation emergency housing and Shanti residences were especially helpful for people on General Assistance. The emergency housing program provides temporary lodgings until a permanent arrangement can be made. These services deal with many difficult problems.

John, for example, a thirty-six-year-old, basically a street person, was admitted to the hospital numerous times. He had KS, pneumocystis, CMV retinitis. He was as impossible as he was endearing. He was not appropriate for Shanti, because he didn't want to give up his drug habit. His SSI check was lost or stolen a couple of times, and he went to the emergency housing each time he was discharged. Finally, a dedicated social worker at the AIDS Foundation helped him secure a subsidized rental that he liked, and after that he settled in.

The Shanti Residence Program has been perhaps unique: It has cooperated with the City and County of San Francisco to make low-cost housing available to persons with AIDS. The city leases units to Shanti Project, which then manages them, and monitors patients in them regularly; additional assistance is provided by community agencies, if required. Because patients live together, networks providing extensive support are established, which often decreases the need for inpatient acute hospital services. In providing inexpensive housing, it has saved many sick persons from being alone and miserable in a downtown hotel room. And, also, I'm sure the program would be in shambles now if it were not managed so beautifully.

A case in point was James: twenty-five years old; first time pneumocystis; young, anxious, frightened. At first he thought he would be able to return to his roommate. But then, because his roommate traveled frequently, and during the course of his treatment he found he was much weaker, much sicker than he'd imagined, he was concerned about being alone so much. He moved into Shanti with help from the AIDS Homecare Program. As with the other organizations, I cannot say enough good things about the AIDS Homecare Program, whose nurses, attendants, and social workers make it possible for people to stay at home. And when Homecare cannot pick up immediately, we do use VNA or public health nurses if less care is needed.

Sometimes when home care is not adequate to the needs of the person, a few extended-care facilities in the Bay Area will take hospice-type patients, usually terminal ones who need a great deal of nursing care, IVs, and oxygen.

One *great* need, however, still, all over the country is for skilled nursing facility convalescent care beds, in cases when a patient is bed-bound, does not need IVs or oxygen, but still needs a lot of good nursing care. In larger geographical areas where patients are few and isolated, regional care centers are also needed.

The kinds of social work I have been describing, in addition to their basic functions, help people with their coping, their motivation, and their strengths—strengths that were so well expressed by Albert Camus: "In the depth of winter I finally learned that within me lay an invincible summer."

19

Coordinated Community-Based AIDS Treatment

HELEN SCHIETINGER

Outlining the range of services needed by and available to persons with AIDS in San Francisco may enable local health professionals to refer clients appropriately and those from other communities to use the information for their own local services.

Let us begin by looking at the historical context. In 1981, in San Francisco, only a handful of people had this disease, which had no name. When I came to the Kaposi's Sarcoma Clinic, the acronym AIDS did not exist. In agencies such as the Hospice of San Francisco services were provided for persons with AIDS, although Medi-Cal and private insurance companies did not cover the cost of their needs.

As the number of AIDS diagnoses increased, it became clear that the health care system could not meet the intense and unique physical and emotional needs of those with AIDS. As public awareness increased, the system also could not address the rising levels of homophobia and fear of contagion among lay people and health care workers alike. New systems had to be developed on a citywide basis to deal with these issues. It was the Department of Public Health, first through Pat Norman's Office of Lesbian and Gay Health, and then through the AIDS Activity Office, which provided the coordination of planning. Essential elements in this planning were to identify and give priority to community needs of those with AIDS in order to make projections of future needs. Future needs identification has been very important in annual budget discussions with the city government and in creating cooperation and communication among potential AIDS service providers. The AIDS Coordinating Committee of the city has met regularly since 1982 in the Department of Public Health. Centralized planning has prevented a duplication of services in the city and assured that existing services are utilized wherever possible. It is important to note that throughout the process we have created liaisons with community services and found allies and advocates within larger systems. There has been a continual attempt to maintain an overview and connection of services within the city.

The other essential element in developing services in this city has been adequate funding. The first two organizations that addressed AIDS were the Shanti Project—an older, well-established organization that provided counseling to people with life-threatening illnesses— and the AIDS Foundation, originally called the KS Foundation—a new community-based organization specifically established to address the AIDS crisis. Both organizations were initially dependent on private donations and, therefore, were low-budget operations. They have been very fortunate that the San Francisco city government recognized the importance of the services provided by these agencies and therefore began funding them both quite early.

Some cities have thought the solution to AIDS was to export anyone diagnosed with the illness. We have provided for many of those exiles because their communities refused to provide care. Other cities have expected volunteers to provide any specialized services needed by persons with AIDS. The services needed *are* specialized and many do not exist within the traditional health care system. But two problems arise from depending solely on volunteers and volunteer organizations to provide the care.

First, many of the needed services are professional, such as home care, mental health care, and social services. Persons with AIDS have a right to be provided these services by the health care system. Second, in order to utilize volunteers it is essential to provide a solid structure, with paid staff to recruit, train, supervise, and support the volunteers. It is not possible to run an organization solely on volunteer energy. This fact is basically important for other communities to recognize in looking at the beginning of their service systems. San Francisco has funded many organizations to provide offices and staff, which then mobilize large numbers of volunteers who do incredibly valuable work.

Structurally, we have seen in San Francisco that providing specialized services for persons with AIDS has augmented the existing mental and physical health care delivery systems, not replaced them, and also that volunteers can be utilized in many ways to enhance the services provided by professionals.

I have identified eight basic areas of specialized services that are needed by persons with AIDS. In 1982 the list would not have been this extensive. But in any service delivery system, the larger the numbers, the more complex and specialized the services will have to be.

The needs were identified and addressed by the city in the order in which they are listed: medical care, emotional support services, information and referral services, housing, social services, home care, substance abuse services, and long-term care. Some providers receive special city funding or are contract agencies of the city.

Medical care is provided by physicians throughout the city. Even though there are specialized services, persons with AIDS do receive services throughout the city in every context within the health care system. The first specialized medical clinic was the KS Clinic at the University of California, San Francisco Medical Center. It has now evolved into the AIDS Clinical Research Center at UCSF.

The next outpatient clinic to develop was the AIDS Clinic at San Francisco General Hospital. This clinic is one of the primary clinics in the country where experimental drug treatment protocols are conducted. The Adult Immunodeficiency Clinic at UCSF also sees and cares for people with AIDS. All hospitals in the city provide AIDS acute and emergency care. At San Francisco General Hospital, the Special Care Unit provides a model for AIDS inpatient care. Here, the care is tailored to meet the emotional and physical needs of the person in much the same way that care is tailored on a renal floor or an oncology floor in a specialized unit. Often, the specialized care units provide a consultation service for the private physician.

As all health professionals involved in AIDS work are aware, emotional support has been critical for persons with AIDS and their support networks for a variety of reasons ranging from public ostracism and homophobia to the grim prognosis of the illness itself. The Shanti Emotional Support Program recruits, trains, supervises, and supports volunteers who provide free counseling to persons with AIDS and their loved ones. Each volunteer has one to three clients and becomes an integral part of the support system of each of them, often spending many hours a week at home or in the hospital with each person. The Shanti Project also conducts support groups for persons with AIDS and their friends, families, and lovers.

Another component of care in San Francisco is pastoral care. Many church groups throughout the city have offered counseling by ministers and by members of their congregations. The AIDS Interfaith Network is a group that represents the diversity of pastoral care in San Francisco.

The Shanti Project provides counselors who staff the AIDS wards at San Francisco General Hospital, helping hospitalized people deal with a range of issues created by their illness—from whether to accept advanced life support to how to tell family members of their diagnosis.

This is a unique program that has truly enhanced the care received by persons with AIDS at San Francisco General Hospital, particularly in assisting them to take more control of their care. One example demonstrates the impact it has made. The Intensive Care Unit at San Francisco General Hospital for a long time was filled with AIDS patients who had been intubated as they went into respiratory distress with *Pneumocystis carinii* pneumonia. But now Shanti counselors assist people when they are first hospitalized to think about whether they want such advanced life support. It has been possible for individuals with AIDS to decide they do not want to be intubated in the event they go into respiratory distress. Thus, the staff knows and is able to act according to the wishes of the individual rather than acting according to standard crisis protocol.

Persons with AIDS often come to the disease with the emotional problems and dysfunctional coping mechanisms that existed before their diagnoses. The community mental health system of the Department of Public Health in San Francisco, Operation Concern, and private clinicians throughout the city provide mental health services. In addition, immediate evaluation and intervention are available for anyone in crisis through the psychiatric social workers and the psychiatrist at the AIDS Clinic at San Francisco General Hospital. These positions are funded through the AIDS Health Project, which directs the major emphasis of its program to the "Worried Well" and to those with ARC, in an attempt to help them develop lifestyles that may prevent them from succumbing to AIDS.

Acute inpatient psychiatric care has been available in the hospital inpatient programs throughout the city. As far as I know, most psychiatric facilities here have dealt with and taken care of AIDS patients as their needs arose.

When the AIDS Foundation was in its embryonic stages, an AIDS hotline was established to provide information and referrals for persons with AIDS, for those who had symptoms or who were frightened of coming down with AIDS, and for those who simply had generalized fears about the disease. The hotline has been a vital first-line service. It directs people to needed services when their anxiety levels may be too high to seek out the resources that are available. This hotline function often gets lost in the more general purpose of the hotline to provide correct information to the public every time a sensational news story breaks. Also, the number of calls that come into the Shanti Project every day has led to the formation of an information and referral department. Originally, there was a deep concern not to create duplication of services in the city, and the hotline and information and referral function was performed only by the AIDS Foundation. Although it is important not to duplicate services, often even specialized organizations may have to reorganize to serve the public needs. This is not duplication, but an extension of needed services.

Housing has been a particularly acute problem for persons with AIDS throughout the country primarily because they face financial devastation when they are unable to work, and also because they face social ostracism resulting from fear of contagion. Many people are banished from their homes by roommates or landlords afraid of catching the disease.

The Shanti Residence Program began in 1982. It provides low-cost permanent housing in small group living situations to people with AIDS who are residents of San Francisco. No direct services are provided to residents of the houses by Shanti. The goal of the program is to enable people whose lives have been disrupted by a diagnosis of AIDS to reassert stability despite the social and financial repercussions of their illness. Although most residents of Shanti houses are independent, many other persons with AIDS have been able to remain in them or their own homes with special care.

A federally funded program for the disabled is one many communities might want to investigate. It is called Section 8 housing, available to anyone with a long-term disability, including AIDS. Long waiting lists, however, do exist for the public housing component, and few private apartments qualify for the subsidy for private housing.

Finally, the AIDS Foundation has an Emergency Housing Program, which provides a temporary haven for persons with AIDS while they look for permanent housing. This has been a critical segment of the service network for people here.

Social services provided by hospitals and home care agencies have been significant in assisting persons with AIDS in applying for local, state, and federal benefits. Very early in the epidemic, however, it became obvious that persons with AIDS fell through the cracks fairly regularly. Many were used to being independent and were ashamed to apply for what they perceived as welfare. Also, the physical and cognitive disabilities of many made it impossible for them to follow through with the completion of applications even when initial forms were filled out by social workers in the hospital. When this problem was identified, a social services department was established at the AIDS Foundation to handle case management. This department created liaisons with bureaucracies such as Social Security, SSI, General Assistance, and the Food Stamp Program; it enabled applications to be processed quickly and sidestepped the resistance of individual offices to deal with AIDS. The social services department of the AIDS Foundation has often handled cases of people who are somewhat socially marginal and who do not fare well in the traditional medical and mental health systems.

The AIDS Fund is a community organization that raises money from private sources and provides limited financial assistance to people with demonstrated need. The Fund has been able to function on a volunteer basis. It is the only organization I know in the city with no paid staff and minimal overhead that has been able to continue to provide its services.

Traditional home care has usually been unable to meet the intense needs of physically disabled persons with AIDS. Home care agencies assume that there is a primary caretaker in the home, and often this is not the case with persons with AIDS. Also, they expect to provide only episodic care during weekly nursing visits, with perhaps periodic personal care provided by a home health aide. But often a person with AIDS becomes dependent both physically and cognitively and requires a greater level of care. Of all the home care agencies that have cared for individuals with AIDS living in Shanti residences, I found that Hospice of San Francisco was the only agency equipped to provide adequate care. And it almost went bankrupt doing so because the services were not reimbursed by enough of the insurance companies and by California's MediCal. So, although most home care agencies in the city do provide limited services to persons with AIDS, the city has funded a special program, the AIDS Home Care and Hospice Unit of the Visiting Nurses Association, which has the comprehensive services usually seen only in an outpatient hospice setting. These services include an on-call registered nurse who is available to people twenty-four hours a day for questions, and an attendant care program that trains its own attendants who provide services in people's homes—not just home health aides who come in for an hour but attendants who spend several hours at a time in service. The program also provides emotional support by staff and trained volunteers, who help deal with issues of illness and of death and dying. It is basically a very comprehensive hospice home care program. It receives a proportion of its funding from the city and also receives third-party reimbursement.

The Shanti Practical Support Program also addresses the physical needs of persons with AIDS who live at home. This program assigns volunteers to individual clients to cook, clean, shop, and do other tasks that the person may need in order to be maintained at home. Each volunteer usually participates four hours a week in this program.

In an outpatient setting, one usually identifies a few people who have apparent alcohol or drug problems. When I began providing housing for people, I found myself much more aware of drug and alcohol problems than I had been in the outpatient clinic setting. In San Francisco, 98 percent of persons with AIDS are gay and bisexual men. We do not have the proportion of heterosexual intravenous drug abusers that are found on the East Coast among persons with AIDS. But 9.8 percent of gay men have admitted to IV drug use. Alcohol and drug abuse exists in epidemic proportions in our society generally as well as in the gay community, and many people we deal with also have diagnoses as substance abusers.

Outpatient treatment has been available for persons with AIDS at Operation Concern and the Haight-Ashbury Drug Program. Also, the Alcohol Evaluation and Treatment Center (AETC) and other inpatient programs throughout the city have provided services to persons with AIDS at one time or another.

But intervention in drug and alcohol abuse in people with life-threatening illnesses is often difficult, both for medical and mental health practitioners. Therefore, the AIDS Substance Abuse Program was developed. It is based at the AIDS Health Project and provides services chiefly at the San Francisco General Hospital AIDS clinic. The program staff is available to assist clinicians in diagnosing and intervening in substance abuse problems among their clients and also to assist persons with AIDS directly in addressing their addictions.

The last area of need to surface in San Francisco has been that of long-term care. So far we have managed either to keep in the hospital persons too debilitated to care for themselves or to maintain them at home with the attendant care provided by the AIDS Home Care Unit. But even this is not designed to provide ongoing care for the person with permanent neurological damage or irreversible physical problems that require round-the-clock care. The AIDS Home Care Unit is not funded sufficiently to provide that kind of attendant care to individuals for months at a time. In the Shanti residences, care has often been provided to two or three people who live in one house, so that attendant care is consolidated and twenty-four-hour coverage is cost-effective. But these are stopgap measures.

In San Francisco we are at the point of needing a subacute long-term facility to provide care for persons with AIDS who have organic brain syndrome and require a structured environment and for those whose intense needs for physical nursing care are ongoing and continuous, but who have no basic acute medical problems that would justify being in an acute-care hospital. I think probably every discharge planner in this city has struggled with the issue of how to discharge someone who actually needs long-term care. A group of us sees the need fairly acutely in our everyday work with persons with AIDS, and we are once again identifying and documenting a need for municipal services to be provided for our clients.

San Francisco has a pretty good track record in establishing needed programs. With much coordination and planning, we have identified real needs and been effective in developing viable programs to meet those needs. The city will doubtless continue to be responsive to efforts to provide services for persons with AIDS.

20

AIDS: Public Policy and Mental Health Issues

STEPHEN MORIN

The California Council on Mental Health is the body that advises the state legislature and the administration on matters related to mental health. The council is very much concerned with the mental health implications of the AIDS epidemic and since 1983 has been advocating an adequate response by the state government to the medical and psychological needs created by this crisis.

AIDS is most frequently understood as a medical phenomenon. Awareness is growing, however, that AIDS has profound psychological ramifications as well. I would like to trace the way in which mental health issues have been handled in the public sector since 1983, and what the future state response might be.

In 1983 the California legislature took two significant actions with regard to AIDS. First, the legislature passed a bill, SB 910 (Roberti), which established the California AIDS Advisory Committee and set up a mechanism for awarding education and information grants throughout the state. The bill included an initial appropriation of $500,000, channeled through the Department of Health Services to fund some of the more innovative programs across the state. In the first year, fifteen projects were funded. This funding was the only money available to many communities, such as San Diego and Santa Barbara.

SB 910 required a great deal of advocacy. In April 1983, on one of my early trips to the state capital to support that bill, I was joined by Gary Walsh, a friend and psychiatric social worker who had been diagnosed with KS in December 1982. We discovered in Sacramento that the legislature knew very little about AIDS. Although AIDS had recently been the cover story in *Newsweek*, more than half of the legislators with whom we met had never heard of AIDS. Gary would often engage the legislators, look them straight in the eye, roll up his shirtsleeve, and show a KS lesion. It was very difficult to ignore him. He would also look at them directly and say that he fully expected to be dead within nine months. In fact, he was. Many legislators became strong supporters of funds for AIDS research as a result of our efforts.

The other major action taken in 1983 was the addition of $2.9 million to the University of California budget for AIDS activities. Deeply concerned about the AIDS crisis, Willie Brown, Speaker of the Assembly, called together researchers from the University of California system trying to determine exactly what would be needed in order to advance their research efforts. As a result, he was able to introduce an allocation in the UC budget. Many of the early breakthroughs in research came from the UC system and were funded through this effort. The discovery of the retrovirus responsible for simian AIDS, for example, was discovered at UC Davis. Later, in Jay Levy's laboratory, at UC San Francisco, a retrovirus responsible for AIDS was isolated. The state funds made possible a number of activities through the UC Task Force on AIDS.

In 1983 California had a budget crisis. Community mental health programs were cut by more than $30 million that year. Governor Deukmejian was adamantly opposed to any new allocations and was specifically opposed to any new allocations for AIDS-related activities. California nevertheless managed to develop a program more elaborate than any developed elsewhere, chiefly because the state legislative leadership supported it. Without Speaker Willie Brown, representing San Francisco, and President *pro tem* of the State Senate, David Roberti, who represents Hollywood, it is very unlikely that California would have any of the programs that currently serve as role models for other states.

A more difficult year was 1984. The major bill, SB 2244 (Roberti), died in committee after strong opposition from the Department of Health Services and the administration. It would have mandated development of a plan for dealing with the AIDS epidemic and would have established the various responsibilities. It would have required coordination of all activities through the health and welfare agency. All that was really accomplished in the 1984 session was a successful effort on the part of Assemblyman Art Agnos (D-San Francisco) and Senator Milton Marks (then R-San Francisco) to double the funds in the information and education grants to a million dollars. The funds allocated through the UC system remained the same.

In marked contrast, the 1985 legislative session involved much activity related to AIDS. Perhaps the most significant of the public policy issues was the passage of AB 488 (Roos). This bill established alternate site testing centers for HIV antibody testing throughout the state

of California. The principal public policy concern leading to this legislation was a desire to protect California's blood supply. During the
months in which this legislation was debated and finally enacted, HIV
antibody testing was licensed by the federal government. This permitted blood banks to screen donor blood for the presence of AIDS antibodies. The legislature was eager to ensure that people who wanted to
know their HIV antibody status be diverted from blood banks as the
sole source of this information. To respond to the legislature's desire,
Assemblyman Roos sponsored a bill that has resulted in innovative and
unique programs in California.

Consider, for example, the mental health aspects of that bill. Armed
with research data from the AIDS Behavioral Research Project at UC
San Francisco, along with staff from the California Council on Mental
Health, I met with Roos's staff and worked out amendments to the bill
to deal with some of the primary mental health issues. The data collected at UCSF revealed that people who were having the antibody
test, or thinking about it, had many misconceptions about what it was
and what it would do.

The council wanted some method of assuring *informed consent* in this
bill, parallel to what is done in mental health with regard to medication. The bill was amended to provide that "at a minimum, individuals
seeking testing shall be informed about the validity and accuracy of the
antibody test before the test is performed. All testing-site personnel
shall be required to attest to having provided the above information."

The second major concern was about the psychological meaning of
the test. The available data indicated that people wanted to be tested
more for *psychological* reasons than for *medical* reasons. Concerned
with what people would do with the information derived from the
test, and particularly what impact it would have on their psychological
well-being, we sought assurances about the means of giving test results. Earlier data indicated that of the people who had been tested
through May 1985, in San Francisco, half had received the results by
telephone. This was similar to a 1983 survey of people with AIDS,
when Walter Batchelor and I found that a large number of tested men
had received their AIDS diagnosis by telephone.

The council asked for amendments, and AB 488 in final form stated
that "all individuals who are tested at the sites established by this article shall be given the results of this test in person."

A third area of concern was the *sensitivity* of personnel at alternate
sites to mental health issues. The bill required specific training in mental health issues. The bill also stated that "all sites providing antibody
testing pursuant to this article shall have a protocol for referral for

twenty-four-hour inpatient mental health services. All individuals awaiting test results and all persons to whom results are reported shall be informed of available crisis services and shall be directly referred, if necessary."

The bill also provided $5 million for alternate site testing programs throughout the state. In yet another brilliant strategy, the bill was double-joined (that is, it could not be enacted unless the latter bill was enacted) to Art Agnos's bill AB 408, which provided for the confidentiality of HIV antibody testing and established penalties for the inappropriate disclosure of the test results. The net effect of these two bills was to establish policies regarding antibody testing in California that are unique and, in their sensitivity to people's well-being, a model for the rest of the country.

It should be noted that mental health services for those who were seropositive were at one time to be funded through this bill. The governor's office threatened a veto of the bill if these provisions were not dropped. Senior staff in his office indicated that Governor Deukmejian did not want to be seen as promoting or condoning *that* life-style. The second major accomplishment of the 1985 legislative session was the establishment of the AIDS Budget Task Force in the legislature. Again this group was called together at the request of Assembly Speaker Willie Brown. The group was chaired by Assemblyman John Vasconcellos of San Jose, chair of the assembly Ways and Means Committee. He is one of the legislators who had listened intently to Gary Walsh in 1983. The Budget Task Force held seven hearings on the immediate budget needs and issued recommendations for an extensive augmentation of the state's AIDS-related efforts, to a sum of $21.5 million.

I testified on mental health issues before the Budget Task Force. The state council had identified many groups, including those people diagnosed with AIDS, as well as their friends, lovers, and families; those with ARC; those who test positive for HIV antibodies; those who suffer from AIDS-related anxiety or somatoform disorders; and those in high-risk groups who suffer from anticipatory or associated distress.

We specifically asked for $5.4 million. We also urged the expenditure of $1 million to train mental health workers in the north and south of the state. Recognizing the limitations within the budget, the Budget Task Force finally ended up allocating $1 million to the Department of Mental Health to be granted to counties for direct mental health services. An additional $1.5 million was placed in the budget for "counseling" associated with AIDS antibody testing. That later had to be changed—we were not permitted to use the word "counseling," which roused the antagonism of the governor's office. It was changed to "preventive education." You can have one hour of preventive education funded through these alternate plans. On June 28, 1985, Governor Deukmejian vetoed *all* the mental health money that was in the budget.

In his veto message the governor indicated that he was eliminating the $1 million augmentation for mental health services to AIDS patients. He indicated that if such services were viewed as a priority by counties they should be funded by the counties.

As part of his veto message he also eliminated $1.5 million for AIDS-related community support services, primarily hospice and home health and attendant care for AIDS patients. The rationale was that there were no data to support the effectiveness and efficiency of such kinds of service. Ironically, at the same time he also vetoed $400,000 in the University of California budget that was targeted for the Institute for Health Policy Studies at UCSF to conduct a study for the legislature on the medical costs associated with AIDS, which would undoubtedly have substantiated the need for the other programs. He also cut $2.3 million for the funding of clinical drug trials of antiviral agents at the UC campuses. In total, the governor vetoed $11.6 million that had been appropriated by the legislature for AIDS-related activities.

Since the governor's veto message the political climate has changed. Rock Hudson has died from AIDS. School children have AIDS. The governor has been strongly lobbied by members of his own party but still is not making AIDS a priority for funding.

As a result of yet another extensive lobbying effort, SB 1251 finally added the $2.3 million back to the university budget in 1985 and included $600,000 for the Department of Mental Health to establish an AIDS Mental Health Project. This money is being used to conduct a statewide assessment of AIDS-related mental health needs. The bill also calls for the state Department of Mental Health to fund education and training of mental health providers throughout the state. The major part of the money, however, is devoted to a media campaign on mental health promotion. The campaign emphasizes basic public information about AIDS—clearly the intent is to reduce some of the irrational fears that have arisen, not only here, but elsewhere around the country. The media campaign is also trying to promote information about the effectiveness of support groups, the relationship between stress and the immune system, and ways of dealing with grief and bereavement.

After more than three years of extensive advocacy, the state of California appears finally to be on the verge of recognizing the psychological aspects of the crisis of AIDS. Much still needs to be done. Particularly, advocacy needs now to be focused on the county level, where direct mental health services are funded. To date, the county of San Francisco has responded admirably to the mental health crisis. Other counties are unlikely to do so unless they receive detailed proposals on the need for such programs.

It is clear that at the state level much advocacy is still needed. The staff in this administration has had little concept until recently of the mental health issues associated with AIDS. We must continue to educate the governor and other state and local policy makers about the reality of AIDS. The last several years at the state level have been difficult. They have been characterized by homophobia and insensitivity to mental health issues. This need not be the case in the future.

Index